Recovering from
THE
HEART ATTACK
EXPERIENCE

BOOKS BY ELIZABETH WEISS:

The Female Breast

Female Fatigue

From Female Depression to Contented Womanhood

The Gourmet's Low Cholesterol Cookbook (with R. Wolfson)

The Cholesterol Counter (with R. Wolfson)

The Protein Planner (with R. Wolfson)

Cookmates (with J. Laskey)

ELIZABETH WEISS

IN COLLABORATION WITH STEPHEN RUBENSTEIN, M.D.

Recovering from

THE

HEART ATTACK

EXPERIENCE

EMOTIONAL FEELINGS · MEDICAL FACTS

Macmillan Publishing Co., Inc.   NEW YORK

Collier Macmillan Publishers   LONDON

Macmillan Publishing Co., Inc.
866 Third Avenue, New York, N.Y. 10022
Collier Macmillan Canada, Ltd.

Library of Congress Cataloging in Publication Data
Weiss, Elizabeth S
   Recovering from the heart attack experience.
   1. Heart—Infarction. 2. Heart—Infarction—
Psychological aspects. I. Rubenstein, Stephen,
joint author. II. Title. III. Title: Heart
attack experience. [DNLM: 1. Coronary disease—
Rehabilitation—Popular works. 2. Coronary
disease—Psychology—Popular works. WG113 W4293r]
RC685.I6W44   616.1'237   80–16719
ISBN 0–02–625830–7

10 9 8 7 6 5 4 3 2 1

Designed by Jack Meserole

Printed in the United States of America

CONTENTS

ACKNOWLEDGMENTS

No cardiologist, no social worker, not even a psychiatrist can know how it really feels to have a heart attack. Only a heart attack victim, his family, and those who care for him can truly understand the tremendous emotional, financial, and personal difficulties. For sharing their thoughts, feelings, and deeply personal experiences, I am indebted to: Sylvia Adler, Estelle Bunin, Norman Bunin, Lynne Bressler, George Davies, Leocadie Davies, Ruth Kirsch, Rochelle McKeever, Gerald Reichenthaler, Ira Reichenthaler, David Schattner, Laura Sacks, Charles Steinberg, and Elias Stoller, M.D.

For providing a personal look at the professional side of cardiac care, I am grateful to Anna Burton, M.D.; Marilyn Citrin, R.N.; Saul Glazer, M.D.; Max Needleman, M.D.; William Nye, M.S.W.; and V. Subramanian, M.D.

In addition, a very special thanks goes to my collaborator, Stephen Rubenstein, M.D., for his conscientious interest and medical expertise; my medical researcher, Miriam Fridman, whose long hours in the library enabled this book to contain the most up-to-date medical findings; and the editor, Toni Lopopolo, whose hard work helped produce this very attractive volume.

And finally, a personal thank-you to my family—my two-year-old and four-year-old sons who had great pride in the fact that "Mommy is a writer," and my husband Stan who, despite family demands, has always insisted that my writing come first.

Why We Wrote This Book

One evening a young editor, extremely upset, telephoned me. Her boss, a vigorous man in his late thirties had suffered a serious heart attack at the office. An avid tennis player, he was "the picture of health." He was married and had two very young children.

When she went looking for a heart book for him, she found many on the biological aspects of heart disease but nothing at all on the emotional ramifications. She asked if I would be interested in writing such a book.

Having just completed a book on depression, I found dealing with feelings fascinating. To assure that the book was absolutely authoritative, I asked Dr. Stephen Rubenstein, a cardiologist at Beth Israel Medical Center in New York City, to collaborate. Together we tried to create a new type of heart book—one that would reflect the very real experiences and emotions of patients and their families as well as the latest medical theories and practices.

We begin the book with feelings—a sampling of scores of interviews with heart attack victims and their families. Their accounts are real; only their names have been fictionalized. Without their experiences, this book would be an empty echo. Their insights provide its inspiration.

Heart attacks happen so suddenly, people function mechanically. Most go through the experience with remarkable success. They return to work; they resume having sex and their depression lifts. But during the weeks between hospitalization and total recovery, there are difficult times, uncomfortable stresses, and often marital strains. No one seems to mention these difficulties which can leave people feeling angry, confused, and isloated.

Because anxiety and depression are often caused by a misunderstanding of the medical problem, Part II of our book is devoted to the medical facts. Today, people are no longer willing to "leave it to the doctor" when a heart problem develops. They are not content with a physician saying only, "George has had a heart attack." They want to know what a heart attack is, why it happened, and what they can do in the future to preserve health and life.

Most importantly, they want the *complete* facts. It is the half-truths, myths, and most of all the unknown that is really frightening and depressing.

Despite all reassurances, it is normal for a person to have a certain amount of anxiety about himself after a heart attack. To a certain extent, this is good, for it acts as a protective mechanism of the body. Overconcern, however, can greatly prolong the convalescence and can lead to an unnecessarily restricted future life. Of course, the return to a normal life is not presented to anyone on a silver platter. It is a difficult task. In this pursuit, many people find a book helpful. By not only informing but also supporting and comforting, we feel this book is special. We hope you will agree.

Questions You May Have

Each hour, 125 men and women in the United States experience heart attacks. This means two heart attacks every minute—day and night. Over one million people suffer heart attacks each year.

Heart attacks occur suddenly and unexpectedly. Not uncommonly, they occur at an early age, such as the mid-forties, even though the highest incidence is in the mid-sixties.

Confusion accompanies heart attacks; worry follows. Victims and their families often have many questions. A physician is the person to ask, but questions often occur when the doctor is not there, or they are forgotten when he is. Some people are reluctant to discuss things fully with their doctor. Even when the most complete guidance is given, instructions can be forgotten.

To speed recovery, it is important that all questions and fears be openly discussed. Following are common questions that victims —the patient, his wife, and his children—ask.

The Patient Asks

Will I lead a normal life again?

Yes. Most patients are able to take up life where they left off, with certain modifications.

How bad is it?

It is impossible to tell immediately the severity of a heart attack. It is possible to have excruciating pain with a mild attack and relatively less pain with a more serious attack. The seriousness of an attack depends on the particular artery that has become blocked, as well as other factors. If it is a major artery—one that carries a large blood supply—then the attack is serious. If the blocked artery is small, then the attack is relatively minor.

A series of tests—electrocardiograms, white-blood-cell counts, and enzyme analysis—will be done. From them, the severity can be determined.

Can I go back to my old job?

It depends on what you did and how you did it. For example, a wallpaper hanger who raises his arms for long periods, a clerk who lifts heavy shipments, or a security guard who climbs stairs may have to switch jobs. Indeed, an insurance agent who leaves his house at 6:00 A.M., drinks seven cups of coffee, and is under a great deal of pressure, might also have to alter his work program. However, studies show most heart attack victims can and do return to their old jobs.

When can I go back to work?

Most patients return to work in two to three months.

Why do I feel so weak and tired?

After a heart attack, most people feel very exhausted. This is not a sign of complication; it is nothing to be alarmed about. Rather, it is an expected part of the recovery which will gradually ease as a person becomes more active.

Can I smoke?

No, never. Cigarette smoking is extremely dangerous for someone who has had a heart attack. A single cigarette can speed up heartbeat and increase blood pressure. Nicotine constricts the blood vessels, which then requires the heart to pump harder for blood and oxygen to circulate throughout the body.

There seems to be somewhat less risk from cigar or pipe smoking, possibly because these are not inhaled.

Can I have a drink when I want one?

This is controversial. Alcohol does affect the heart. It can predispose even the normal heart to extra beats. It can also seriously affect any medicine you may be taking.

In uncomplicated cases, a social drink on occasion is acceptable. Beer or wine are better than hard liquor.

Do I have to take medicines for the rest of my life?

It varies. Some patients go home from the hospital without medications and never need them. Others go home with some medicine and remain on it indefinitely. If you are given medicine, it should not interfere with the resumption of a normal lifestyle. However, it is imperative that you follow your doctor's instructions carefully.

When can I drive again?

Driving requires little energy, but it does cause stress. Most people can drive after about five weeks. If you have to drive in heavy traffic or for long distances or in very hot or very cold areas, it might be best to wait longer—ten to twelve weeks. Again, check with your doctor first.

Will I have a lot of pain?

Most patients have no pain at all.

Does pain mean I am having another heart attack?

Not usually. After a heart attack, some patients do have chest pain. This pain may be angina pectoris (*angina* meaning constricting pain, *pectoris* meaning chest). It is usually a brief pain, brought on by physical exertion, intense emotion, or eating a heavy meal, and is relieved by rest or a drug called nitroglycerin. It occurs when the heart is receiving too little blood and oxygen.

Pain is a warning sign. If you feel any pain—particularly pain while at rest or long-lasting pain—notify your doctor *immediately*.

Can we have sex?

This is often the first question a person asks.

You *can* have sex; in fact you probably should. Sex can relieve tension: Sexual abstinence may cause strain.

Sexual activity should be resumed slowly, usually about three to eight weeks after an attack. Ultimately a person should be able to return to his or her previous frequency and intensity of sexual activity. A man or a woman after a heart attack can have orgasms.

You may have heard stories of men having heart attacks during intercourse. Sexual relations with a spouse or usual partner are about as strenuous as briskly climbing two flights of stairs. It can almost always be tolerated without any real danger. However, extramarital sex, particularly with a much younger partner in unfamiliar surroundings, *has* been associated with cardiac complications and is dangerous.

You should wait at least two hours after a meal before sexual intercourse. You should not have sex when you are over-tired. Many doctors recommend the woman taking the dominant position, but this is not always necessary. Your physician will be able to give you specific advice.

Is there anything I should not *do?*

Absolutely. I call them the "drastic don'ts":

· don't shovel snow
· don't run after anything
· don't exert yourself immediately after a meal: rest at least one half hour
· don't carry luggage—even a few hundred yards to a taxi
· don't change a tire, no matter what
· don't try to prove to yourself that you are as good as you used to be. Don't play two hours of singles tennis in 90° heat or take on a teenager in basketball.

Your doctor has told you your physical and emotional limits. Don't exceed them!

The Wife Asks

How should I treat him?

A wife should be understanding but she shouldn't treat her husband like a baby. A heart attack need not and should not make a man an invalid. A wife should lead the way back to a normal life.

What can I make him to eat?

Most doctors will give you a no-salt-added, low-cholesterol diet upon discharge from the hospital.

Can we go to a restaurant?

Certainly. A patient usually stays around the house for the first few weeks. But about the time he returns to work—generally two months after an attack—he can dine out.

Can I use salt in cooking?

No, salt should not be used in cooking or at the table. In a normal diet, people eat about eight to nine grams of salt per day; a heart patient should eat about three to four grams. Again, cases vary, so check with your doctor.

Can he help me around the house when he's recovering?

Why not? He shouldn't be lifting laundry, pushing a broom, or polishing furniture. But he can certainly make a bed, dust, or set the table. If he feels tired, he should stop immediately.

Can we have company?

Of course. Don't have someone who will provoke an argument. And don't become overfatigued.

Can we go on vacation?

Not right away, but three to four months after an attack, you probably can. In fact, you probably should.

You can travel by plane without problems.

If you travel by car as a passenger, stop often, get out and walk around. This will prevent blood clots in the legs. Under no circumstances should you carry your luggage. Take an adequate supply of medicine with you.

The Children Ask

When will Daddy be home?

Your Daddy will probably stay in the hospital twenty-one days.

When can Daddy play?

He can play as soon as he gets home. At first, try to select some special "quiet time" things. He can certainly read you a story, do a puzzle, even go for a walk. Eventually, he can probably throw a baseball, even play a game of tennis doubles, but these will have to wait until the doctor gives the go-ahead.

Can we make noise around the house?

Certainly. You can and should live normally, but be considerate. If Daddy wants to nap, be quiet.

Is my Daddy going to die?

There is every reason to believe Daddy will become completely well again. He may be on a diet, take more or less exercise, and go to bed a little earlier. In most cases, however, Daddy will go back to his normal life.

You probably have other questions. Most people are worried and concerned after a heart attack. Few just shrug it off—take it in stride.

Being informed is essential. If you have had a heart attack already, it is important to know what activities place excessive demands on the heart and should be avoided. It is equally important to know what you can and should continue to enjoy without fear or anxiety.

Even if you have never had a heart attack, awareness is extremely important. Untold millions of men and women are right on the brink—sitting ducks for heart attacks. These people who may momentarily join the ranks of the coronary population should know that heart disease is not inevitable. They can and should decrease their risk of heart disease.

Recovering from the Heart Attack Experience is not for men only. While men are much more prone to heart attacks, women are hardly immune.* Indeed, since women are exposing themselves to the stresses of competitive business, they are suffering more heart attacks.

This book is for young and old alike. Although the risk of a heart attack increases with age, the time to prevent it is when you are young. Eating habits and smoking begin early. Forming healthy habits at a young age can pay lifesaving dividends later on.

---

* It should be noted here that the use of "he," "his," etc. in this book refers to all heart patients, male *and* female.

A heart attack is not just a medical problem; it is an emotional crisis as well. Not only the victim but family and friends must make psychological adjustments. So here is the whole story—the emotional feelings that no one ever discusses as well as the medical facts.

PART ONE

Emotional Feelings

I. "I Had a Heart Attack"

A HEART ATTACK is an intensely personal experience. "You cannot live until you have almost died," one heart victim told us. "It taught me life is too short to be mad at anybody," a fifty-year-old woman said. Although each person's experience and reactions are unique, by reading the experience of others, perhaps you will recognize portions of your own. This will not only be comforting, it will also be informative. It will show you life is not about to end; you will not become a semi-invalid.

A heart attack can happen to anyone—young or old, rich or poor, athlete or sedentary individual. We spoke with scores of victims whose ages, economic status, and symptoms varied widely. However, their feelings and personal ruminations were startlingly similar. Here are just a few of their stories as they told them:

Jacob Silver is a fifty-three-year-old gastroenterologist. He is married for the second time and has three sons. On June 26, 1976, Dr. Silver suffered a severe myocardial infarction. "I celebrate the date each year as my second birthday," he told us. Today Dr. Silver maintains a full work schedule, a normal social life, and jogs three miles daily.

"I had finished my rounds on a Saturday morning and went to play tennis. We played to a six-to-six tie on a grueling hot day. Then I sat around the club pool, read the *Times*, and went into the sauna. I didn't stay long. As I walked out, I began to feel nauseated, and decided to get dressed quickly.

"Next thing I knew I passed out. I never had any chest pain, but was very, very nauseated.

"I tried to get up and dressed but wound up flat on my back again with faces looking at me. Then I broke into a terrific sweat and had terrific cramps. I had to get to the bathroom in the worst way and started toward the bathroom. Then I was down again.

"I heard someone say 'Do whatever you have to do here.' I had a terrific defecation in a blanket.

"Someone called an ambulance; it came and picked me up. I was completely nude, just wrapped in a blanket.

"They slammed the ambulance door on my big right toe. It was still black and blue six months later, but it gave me a jolt. At least, I knew I was still alive.

"They wheeled me into the emergency room. I remember being on the stretcher, seeing all those bright lights in the hospital ceiling, and passing light after light. They put me into a cubby, and started to work on me.

"I felt like I wasn't there. I heard everything, but I didn't feel like I was part of it. I was sort of up on top of the stretcher. I heard 'Give him another shot—his rate is 32.' Nothing hurt. I had a temporary pacemaker put in, then I was wheeled up to the Coronary Care Unit. I think I slept through the first day.

"When I was lying on the floor I remember thinking, 'You know this is the way you're going to die with no one you know around.' I was thinking mainly of my sons.

"At the time, it wasn't a frightening experience; I wasn't hysterical. I was white and clammy-looking. But I was calm. I couldn't speak, though. I knew the words but couldn't transport them through my vocal apparatus. I opened my mouth to speak but no words came out.

"Interestingly enough, I didn't realize what was happening. I'm fairly intelligent, a better than average doctor, but I never thought I was having a heart attack. It just never dawned on me.

"I spent the next four or five days in the CCU. From the first day, I never had any pain or discomfort. In fact in all the three years since the initial attack, I've never had a single pain.

"Interestingly, the day I was admitted three other young guys were admitted. All had been taken off tennis courts. At fifty, I was the oldest; one guy was thirty-five.

"After a week in the CCU, I went to a semiprivate room. A seventy-nine-year-old man with his third heart attack was there. He pulled out a huge cigar and said 'What the hell difference does it make!'

"Throughout the course of my entire coronary, I never was scared. I just didn't give a damn.

"My sons were on my mind and I thought a lot about my late wife. Eventually, I transferred to a private room. One day I had a terrific crying spell when thinking of my sons. They weren't with me; one was in California and he was having problems. My first wife was something very special. We were married twenty-eight years before she died, and I don't think I ever got over her death. I cried like a baby. After that, I felt better.

"Gradually, I began to wash and shave. As time went on, I'd walk visitors back to the elevator. I was in the hospital four weeks. They kept me an extra week because I was a doctor and they were worried I'd rush things.

"My brother drove me home. I had to pay the bill before I left; I gave the hospital a check. They took me out in a wheelchair. I had lost fifteen pounds and I was drawn-looking. When I left the hospital, they assured me I would be back in full action with no restrictions.

"I left the hospital with mixed feelings. I was anxious to get home, but I wasn't sure if I'd be able to do things.

"At home, I wasn't myself. I began to withdraw, to feel I was less than the rest of the world. When I went out, I wouldn't carry my wallet; I wanted to be non-identifiable.

"The depression hit practically the first day home and lasted a month or two. I was washed out. I felt a hell of a lot better in the hospital. I stayed home about two months. Every afternoon I took a two to three hour nap.

"What helped me get out of it? Working! When I got in the car I'd forget; during the day I'd lose myself in my work.

"About September I went back to work. I also began testing myself by walking around the block twice. I'd pick up speed, then I'd walk a little further. I have a big terrace. I started to jog on my terrace.

"I don't think I really changed from the experience. Doctors tell you to change your ways, but there's no way to change your ways. You are what you are. I think it did make me more cynical about material things—paintings, china, clothes. Who cares?

"And I think it made me a much better doctor. It gives you a tremendous perception to be on the other side of the chart. We're used to giving orders, not taking them. It puts things in a much different focus."

George Wilson is a forty-eight-year-old building superintendent. He is married and has three children. He is back at work full-time, although he still tires more easily. Mr. Wilson finds "I have a different attitude toward life now. I don't want to take any abuse, and in my line of work, you get a lot of abuse. I just don't have the patience I used to."

"It happened sort of fast. For a year or two, I had pain in my arm—I thought it was arthritis. I had been a milkman for many years, out seven days a week, in the cold. Finally, I went to the doctor. He took an EKG and recommended a heart specialist who put me in the hospital. While they were admitting me, the pain seemed to disappear, and I had no pain until I was coming home. I got in a cab and had pain again. I came home but the pain just wouldn't quit. I took ten nitroglycerin but it didn't go away.

"What was the pain like? There was severe pain in the left arm and chest. I thought it was indigestion but it wouldn't go away. I lay down; I sat up; nothing helped.

"So they put me back in the hospital and ran some tests. They suggested an angiogram. That's how they found I had two blocked arteries. They suggested I have bypass surgery. It came as a shock; I never expected it.

"But the surgery wasn't as bad as I expected. Four weeks after the operation I was back at work. I'd say life was back to normal in two months."

Chuck Lothrop is a sixty-year-old trial attorney. He is married, has two daughters and a granddaughter. Chuck suffered his first heart attack at age forty-five, his second at fifty-five.

"My heart attack was at the best place possible—a bar mitzvah. There's got to be a doctor there.

"After the bar mitzvah we had a few drinks, a real good lunch, and then we were dancing the hora.

"All of a sudden, I had this cold clammy feeling, as though some big guy had his arm down my throat and he was twisting. I ran into the men's room where I got very, very violently ill. I have never been that nauseated in my entire life. It felt like I had something coming out of every orifice, including my ears.

"My wife came looking for me. She found me and I was still sick; they stretched me out on the floor. A doctor came and asked me about the pain. My extremities started to get numb.

"This was Saturday and it was Memorial Day. The doctor phoned another doctor who lived nearby, and we drove over to his house. He was in the midst of a picnic and came out in a big chef's hat. He gave me a shot of Demerol and made arrangements at the hospital so when we got there, they were waiting for me. By then, it was three or four o'clock.

"After that, I blanked out. When I came to, it was Tuesday or Wednesday. They placed me on absolute bed rest for about six weeks. I couldn't even watch television 'cause it was too stressful. In fact, I wasn't even allowed to speak.

"I was very unhappy. The doctor could see it, so he asked how he could help. I said I'd like a cigarette. He said, 'You can have a cigarette, in fact, you can smoke all you like. You just have to decide one thing—you can smoke or you can live. Which is it?'

"Then he asked if there was any other way he could help. I said I'd like a drink. He said, 'Absolutely.' He gave my wife permission and told the staff that I would be having liquor. Every day at 4:00 P.M. like clockwork, the nurse ceremoniously poured me half an ounce of Scotch. At first, I wasn't even allowed to hold the glass; I had to take it through a straw. But that became our four o'clock cocktail hour for my entire stay.

"After I got out of the hospital and was allowed to take a walk, I remember I stole a cigarette from my wife's purse. I sat down where no one could see me and lit up. It tasted so awful I snuffed it out, and I haven't had a cigarette since. Before that I was a three-packs-a-day man.

"Giving up smoking didn't bother me. The diet didn't bother me. I think the physical adjustment is easy; it's the mental adjustment that's tough.

"Living with the threat of sudden death is difficult. Conquering fear is essential—you can't just say 'Fear, fear go away, come again another day.' You have to make a conscious effort to dissipate it. If you wake up in the middle of the night with a gas pain or even an imaginary pain, you wonder, is this the time? If you let that type of thinking get to you, you can go mad. You have to realize that life itself is a terminal illness, and you're getting closer to the end, no matter what.

"For me, the key has been putting problems in their proper perspective. Before these episodes, I didn't always do that. Now I think there are no insoluble problems—Every problem has a solution. Today, I focus on the solution, not the magnitude of the problem."

David Kay is a handsome, bearded, virile thirty-three-year-old graduate accounting student. He had his first heart attack at age thirty-two; his second three months later. He has two children, ten and eight, is married for the second time, and lives in Soho.

"I had just gotten to work. I was barely in the door when I got a terrible backache. I said to my boss, 'Give me a big hug and press my back.' She started to, but I began to sweat through two shirts and a baseball warm-up jacket. You could have wrung them out; my hair was soaking.

"To myself, I said, 'This is not "going home" sick, this is "going to hospital" sick.' I was on the verge of passing out and I had terrible chest pain. They rushed me in a taxi to the hospital.

"I've never felt that sick before. All I wanted was the strongest painkiller they had, but I had to wait two and a half hours before they got to me. I tried to move around to get a little relief. It helped a little but not much. I had no idea it was a heart attack. I didn't know what it was—I just knew I had never been that sick.

"Finally, they got to me. I was annoyed because they were taking care of drunks first. Talk about efficiency! When they examined me, I heard one doctor say to another, 'Idiot, he's having a heart attack!' I was sent upstairs to intensive care, spent a week there, and then two weeks on the floor. Most of the time in the hospital I wasn't worried about my condition. It just hadn't sunk in. I knew I was sick, but I figured it would go away.

"The hospital wasn't bad; there were always people around. In fact, I felt lonely when I left at first. It didn't bother me at all to be the youngest on the floor—age didn't seem to matter. Some of those guys couldn't move at all. There were some really sick people there, and it made me realize that everyone has problems.

"The first week home was okay. I had to stay indoors, so I read a little. Then I couldn't read anymore, but I had hopes of being up and out soon. By the end of the second week, I was feeling guilty, and it seems with time, things have gotten worse, much worse.

"I'm very sexually aggressive. Before this I'd have sex five times a week or more. The doctor told me to wait three weeks. I did, but then I couldn't perform. I started feeling very guilty and was afraid of having that pain again. I started to get fed up. I want to be the provider and I'm not. I want to be the man sexually, and I'm not.

"I've taken on the role of housewife, but sometimes I can't get myself to do it. Last week, my wife worked the whole day and then I didn't buy food so we didn't have anything to eat when she came home. She was annoyed, but I just couldn't do it. I feel bad when she has to clean the apartment after working all day, yet I feel lousy being the housewife.

"I'm angry, but I can't get my anger out. I keep everything bottled up inside.

"I hate when people help me and I tell them to get off my back. I don't need mothers. I'm a proud person—if I need help, I ask for it; I don't hesitate a bit. But I can't stand people babying me.

"My wife and I are breaking up. I'm sort of initiating it. The relationship is falling apart; I've got to get away to do some things and I need time for myself. Both of us are pretty confused, I guess.

"Help? We've received none, nothing. In the hospital, we saw a film on Joe Schmo who was mowing his lawn. It was ridiculous —the guy was sixty—it had nothing to do with me.

"Sure I ask 'Why me?' But it's in the family. My grandfather died at fifty of a heart attack; my father also died at fifty of a heart attack. Both were heavy smokers. My dad went to work two weeks after his attack and died at the railroad station.

"When I was in the hospital, I looked back at what I was doing. During the summer, I had been working long hours in a restaurant, always on my feet. I wondered if the job might have brought it on. Maybe I shouldn't have done it, but what should I do? What can I do?

"In the hospital I saw a lot of anger on the part of the patients;

I couldn't blame them. They'd be nasty to their wives—not want to see them. The spouses seemed very reasonable; they loved them or felt sorry for them—or a little bit of both.

"I wish I had someone to talk to. The psychologist I'm seeing now hasn't been through it. I'd like to get into a cardiac club. I guess my feelings are the same as older guys. I feel I'm no good anymore."

All these accounts would be little more than curiosities if only an occasional person fell victim to a heart attack. But today, heart attacks are becoming epidemic. They are the leading killer of middle-age American men.

Stark Statistics

One out of every five Americans has heart disease. The resulting physical, mental, and economic suffering of individuals and their families is so enormous it cannot even be measured. It is horrifying to realize that during the entire ten years of the Vietnam war, the number of people killed was less than 20 percent of the casualties from heart disease in the U.S. in one year alone!

Stark statistics show about 20 percent of all victims die after a heart attack. Another 10 to 20 percent suffer some permanent discomfort and have to adjust their lifestyle. Well over two-thirds of all heart attack victims return to a near normal life.

The peak years for male heart attacks are in the fifty-five to fifty-nine age bracket. The percentage of deaths from first heart attacks is highest among men in their forties however. Doctors believe this is because younger men do not have as well-developed collateral circulation.

Is It a Heart Attack?

As you can see from these actual case histories, symptoms of a heart attack vary widely. Those who experience it cannot always describe what they feel but they know it is extremely serious. Even when there are few other symptoms, that sense of doom is there. The commonest symptoms of a heart attack include:

· chest pain—a pressure that varies from oppressive pain to a squeezing
· radiating pain—in the neck, jaw, right or left shoulder, arm, or between the shoulders in the back
· excessive cold, clammy sweating
· a grayness in the face
· nauseousness, vomiting
· great anxiety
· shortness of breath
· difficult breathing

What Should You Do If You Think You Are Having a Heart Attack?

Take no chances—get help immediately. Go to a hospital any way you can as fast as you can.

Suppose it's the middle of the night? It doesn't matter. Get help fast. People brought to the hospital by ambulance or car immediately after they feel the attack stand a far better chance of surviving than those who wait. In some cases, a few minutes can mean the difference between life and death.

Why Immediate Help Is So Important

Immediate medical attention after a heart attack can save lives.

In most heart attacks—some say almost 85 percent—the damage to the heart muscle is not enough to cause death. Most people die because damage to the heart muscle upsets the heart rhythm. There can be very rapid beating of the ventricles, the heart's pumping chamber. In a short time, that kind of beating can turn into ventricular fibrillation—a useless twitching or quivering—instead of beating. This leads to cardiac arrest, or complete failure of the heart to pump blood.

All of these disturbances can be treated successfully, if treated in time. But these problems usually happen early in a heart attack, before people get to the hospital.

Over 300,000 people die of heart attacks each year before getting to the hospital. Most deaths occur in the first few hours after the attack. Indeed, over 25 percent die within three hours after the onset of their first heart attack.

This is tragic because in hospitals both wild beating and heart stoppage can be controlled. Electric shock (via defibrillator paddles) applied to the person's chest can change irregular beating to regular beating.

When University of Rochester cardiologists did a special study to find out how much time had elapsed between the onset of symptoms and hospitalization, the average interval turned out to be three and a half hours. In some cases, the delay stretched for as long as five days. Transportation to the hospital accounted for only a tiny fraction of the delay—twenty minutes on average. The trouble was that people were slow to seek help even when symptoms should have been unmistakable. Eighty percent had intense chest pain, yet they delayed seeking help.

Studies have shown that older people wait longer than young people. People delay longer when they're alone than when they're with somebody. And taking over-the-counter medicine for what you may believe is indigestion causes further delay.

Undoubtedly, the most important and urgent message in this book is GET HELP IMMEDIATELY if you suspect you are having a heart attack.

An Emotional Event

After a heart attack, everyone—regardless of age, sex, or economic status—goes through certain predictable emotional phases. As Stephan Lesher, who relives his own heart attack at age thirty-eight in his book *A Coronary Event*, describes:

Nancy would visit clad in her tennis dress and when she left my good-bye smile would turn to tears with the speed of a quick-change artist. I resented my inability to join the tennis. . . . Worse, I resented the people who *could* play tennis. And especially, I resented those who could prevent me from doing so. I was acting like a spoiled child, but I couldn't seem to help myself. I was mentally stamping my foot so that everyone's attention would be focused on me—and worse, I thought I deserved it.

Much later, one doctor told me that I had followed the classic pattern of heart patients. Fear of death would turn to anxiety over returning to a normal life but that would lead to depression and the assumption that life would never be the same.

Finally, heart patients tend simply to reject the notion of being sick at all. I don't know if it would have changed anything but perhaps it would have eased my mind to have been told in advance to expect my emotions to bounce around like a rubber ball.

These emotional phases are:

PHASE I.   *Shock and Disbelief*

Immediately following a heart attack, a person experiences a stunned numbness due to the suddenness of the attack. This phase is generally short-lived (usually from twenty-four to forty-eight hours) and is characterized primarily by two behavioral responses —anxiety and denial. For example, although Dr. Silver had treated heart attacks for years, denial was so strong he didn't even recognize his own coronary.

PHASE II.   *Developing Awareness*

This usually begins after the first forty-eight hours, when the shock wears off. After the first night, the person starts to feel better and then frequently denies he ever had a heart attack. Then about the third day, his imagination starts working. He conjures up every possible catastrophic complication. These fantasies often lead to depression.

During this time, the person will also undergo regression. Because he is treated like a child—fed, washed, and helped with all bodily functions—he will become very dependent. As he becomes more aware and feels better, he will be torn between dependence and independence.

PHASE III.   *Resolution*

The last phase, and perhaps the most difficult, begins when the patient leaves the hospital. Then the person must deal with the consequences of his heart attack. Depression, fear, hostility, anxiety, and denial are experienced in various intensities.

Practical Tips for Getting Back

A heart attack is a major life event. It cannot be ignored, but one must not over-exaggerate its importance. Becoming a psychological cardiac cripple is many times more damaging than the actual physical damage to heart muscle. To lead a health-minded but normal life after a heart attack, here are some quick, practical, personal tips:

1. Always carry your medicine with you.
2. Keep an extra supply of nitroglycerin in the house in case of emergency.
3. Fold up an EKG and keep it in your wallet at all times.
4. Take a half-hour's walk outside each day.
5. Tape to your telephone (or nearby) the number of your physician, your closest hospital emergency room, ambulance services, and all-night taxi service.
6. Get out of bed gradually. (Getting out quickly can cause dizziness and fainting.)
7. Never shovel snow.
8. If you feel stressed, stop, close your eyes, breathe deeply three times, and make a conscious effort to relax.
9. Never overeat.
10. Don't strain when constipated if you can help it. (If you must, be sure to keep your mouth open.)
11. Don't put off a needed vacation.
12. Don't diagnose or treat yourself. Never take another heart patient's medicine. (It can be fatal; it is also a violation of state and federal law.)
13. Don't exert yourself immediately after a meal; rest at least half an hour.
14. If caught in an air terminal or railway station with two heavy bags and no porter, don't risk the heart strain of carrying them a few hundred yards to a taxi.
15. Don't fill up on a "fat" snack before bedtime.

16. If you get a flat tire at midnight on a lonely country road, don't change it. If you can't get help, determine to sleep right where you are until morning.

17. When you leave your house on a cold day, cover your mouth and nose with a handkerchief or scarf until you get accustomed to the cold.

18. Get dressed every day.

19. Don't sacrifice sex. It's important and needed for both health and happiness.

20. Don't stay fat. Being fat aggravates diabetes, high blood pressure, coronary disease, kidney diseases, and stroke. And it's unattractive.

21. Don't be fatalistic and say, "There's nothing anyone can do for heart trouble; when your number is up, it's up!" Constant good care—from the physician, from the family, but first and foremost from yourself—is the most important factor in long life and good health.

22. Don't try to prove to yourself that you are as good as you used to be. Don't play seventy-two holes of golf on a weekend or take on a teenager for five sets of tennis singles. Never over-exercise.

23. Consciously try to enjoy each day. Think positively.

24. See your doctor periodically even though you feel fine.

25. Worry less. All people worry. But those who make a conscious effort to be optimistic will live longest (and be happiest)!

2. Common Worries: Myths and Realities

MYTHS are powerful; they can psychologically cripple. Men can become impotent if they fear sexual intercourse after a heart attack. A life of dread and fear may be led if a person believes another heart attack is inevitable.

Nothing is black or white, especially for heart attack victims. Moderation is the key. By separating myth from reality, you and your family can better understand your condition and its proper treatment.

MYTH #1: *"It won't happen to me."*

"I never expected it. Of course, I'm overweight, and I smoke. Yes, I'm under tremendous pressure. But I was always healthy as an ox. I never thought it would happen to me," recalled one man shortly after his attack. Most people think disease only happens to others. Unfortunately one person out of every five gets heart disease.

Certain people are more likely to get heart disease than others. The more of the risk factors you have the more likely you are to have a heart attack. The risk factors are:

- family history of heart attacks at an early age
- high blood pressure
- high blood lipid levels
- smoking
- diabetes
- an overly competitive, aggressive, impatient personality
- overweight
- physical inactivity
- stress
- high uric acid levels

Exactly how to reduce your risk factors so it *doesn't* happen to you will be discussed in the following chapters.

MYTH #2: *Only high-level executives or people under the stress of intensive business competition get heart attacks.*

Heart attacks are *not* the exclusive privilege of company presidents and top executives. There is a false stereotype that the higher the position, the greater the stress, and thus the greater the risk of a heart attack. Heart attacks hit at every level on the social scale almost equally from managers to blue collar workers.

Indeed, many studies show that those with college educations and those successful in achieving their goals have fewer heart attacks than less educated and less successful individuals. Apparently the less educated have to work harder and under greater stress to achieve and hold their jobs.

One study of a hundred young coronary patients found that at the time of their heart attacks ninety-one of these men were holding down two jobs, working more than sixty hours a week, or experiencing unusual fear, insecurity, discontent, frustration, restlessness, or feelings of inadequacy in connection with their work.

A large-scale study covering 270,000 men employed by the Bell System studied men of different job levels. The study failed to find that men with greater responsibility had any more risk of heart attack than those with lesser responsibility.

MYTH #3: *Only men get heart attacks.*

Heart attacks *are* more frequent in men. Women are protected by their sex hormones, or "hormonal shield," as doctors call it.

Heart attacks are rare in normally menstruating women. After menopause (whether natural or artificial) the heart attack rate in women increases.

Up to age forty-five, men have thirteen times as many attacks as women. From forty-five to sixty-two, men have twice as many attacks. After age sixty-two women are just as susceptible as men.

Heart disease causes more than 200,000 deaths a year among American women. That's 60 percent more than die from cancer. Women who smoke or use oral contraceptives have a much greater risk of having a heart attack. In fact, the heart attack incidence in young women who smoke and also use birth control pills is astonishingly high.

Today, with women returning to the business world, they are becoming more cardiac prone. Recent studies show that women who feel they're under constant pressure to adhere to time schedules are two to three times more likely to have heart attacks than women who are more relaxed and easygoing.

MYTH# 4: *Heredity plays such an overwhelming role in heart disease that no action can ever change a person's predisposition to develop heart disease.*

If one or both of your parents, your brothers or sisters, or one or both of your grandparents had heart attacks at early ages, the odds are greater that you will have a similar experience *unless you do something to reduce them.* It is *not* simply a matter of fate. It can be very much a matter of environment.

The exact roles of heredity and environment cannot be clearly separated. Is an obese person that way because of eating habits or is the trait genetically transferred? Generally, it is believed that obesity isn't in the genes, but is due to eating habits developed in childhood. Children of smoking parents are far more likely to smoke than the children of nonsmoking parents. Smoking is not in the genes—it is a matter of environment.

Often the same is true for heart disease. There may be hereditary predispositions for these problems, but the predispositions needn't invariably and inevitably lead to actualities. You may not develop high cholesterol if certain environmental influences are changed so they differ from those acting on other members of your family.

Tests have shown that people who begin to take care of themselves early in life have many more years free of heart trouble than those who ignore the risk factors. And attacks, if they do happen, are less severe and recovery chances are greater.

MYTH #5: *I would certainly know if I had a heart attack.*

"I had no idea," one business executive recalled. "I thought it was indigestion." (Probably half of the people who have a heart attack mistake it for indigestion.)

"Personally, I didn't think he was having a heart attack," his wife admitted. "He didn't look it; his color was good. He wasn't perspiring or short of breath."

A heart attack may cause severe pain in the chest. "It's not really a pain," a heart attack victim explained. "It's pressure. It felt like a vise was tightening across my upper torso—it's a feeling I'll never forget."

Not all chest pain or pressure means a heart attack. Other conditions can produce this type of chest pain. Gallbladder disease can produce pain in the chest. Pleurisy, an inflammation of the lining of the lungs, can cause this type of pain. Shingles, a disease in which the nerves become infected, can cause similar pain. Ulcers in the stomach or duodenum can produce a burning pain. (This is relieved by milk or antacid.)

A hiatus hernia—a condition in which part of the stomach may protrude up through an enlargement in the diaphragm—can be mistaken for a heart attack. Hernia pain usually starts sometime after a person has gone to bed after a large meal. Most people find they get relief if they sit up in bed or get up and walk around. (A hiatus hernia can be seen on an X ray and treated.)

Chest pain can also be due to shoulder bursitis, particularly when the left shoulder is affected. An unsuspected broken rib, which may have happened during a bout of coughing, can cause chest pain. And not uncommonly, excessive air swallowing may account for worrisome chest pain. An episode of food poisoning might cause this kind of discomfort.

About 20 percent of people who have a heart attack are totally unaware of it. These "silent" coronaries can be seen on electro-cardiograms. They occur without symptoms—often in diabetics because their nerves often do not sense the pain as blood vessels close off gradually over a period of weeks or months rather than suddenly over a period of minutes or hours.

Indeed, doctors cannot always tell just by examining a patient if they are having a heart attack. When doctors put their stethoscope over the chest they ask themselves questions such as: Are the heart sounds muffled? Is the rhythm irregular?

Final diagnosis usually depends on technology. In a heart attack, enzymes called CPK, SGOT, and LDH leak from the dying cells into the blood. Results of blood samples taken twenty-four hours after a heart attack, may show these enzyme changes. After a heart attack, the enzymes usually rise sharply and then drop almost as fast. Evidence of a heart attack is also apparent on electrocardiogram tracings.

MYTH #6: *A heart attack is caused by a clot in the coronary artery.*

Although heart attacks are alarmingly common, they are still one of the most puzzling disorders in modern medicine. Doctors understand them partly at best.

Traditional belief held that a clot forms in an artery that is already narrowed by deposits of fatty substances. The clot closes off the blood supply, depriving an area of the heart of sufficient oxygen. This causes death of a portion of the heart muscle.

However, recent studies in Sweden have shown that the clot may follow, rather than precede many heart attacks. These studies reveal that a section of the heart had already begun to die before the clot formed.

Another current theory is that heart attacks are due to spasms of the muscle in the wall of an otherwise normal coronary artery or in a narrowed artery. Research is continuing. More and more the culprit or "the clot" is being questioned.

MYTH #7: *People who have heart attacks have abnormally high cholesterol levels in their blood.*

Yes, cholesterol does contribute to arteriosclerosis. And, yes, abnormally high cholesterol and triglyceride levels do increase your risk of having a heart attack. But people with normal and below normal cholesterol levels can and do have heart attacks.

The average normal American male has a cholesterol level of under 250 mgm. Men with cholesterol levels over this should make an effort to cut their cholesterol.

Some people cannot understand why even when they reduce the cholesterol in their diet, their cholesterol levels remain high. Cholesterol comes from two sources:

1. *Extrinsic:* from the foods we eat.
2. *Intrinsic:* cholesterol is made by the body.

All of us make cholesterol but some people manufacture more than others. Some people are born with a gene which causes them to mass-produce cholesterol.

Luckily, cholesterol is only one of the many risk factors and it is one that can be controlled.

MYTH #8: *A sudden insult to the heart is a heart attack.*

A heart attack is just one of many things that can go wrong with the heart. While many people mistakenly call any heart problem a heart attack, doctors reserve the term for a specific condition—the sudden death of a portion of the muscle that makes up the heart.

Physicians have other names for heart attack: coronary occlusion, coronary thrombosis, myocardial infarction. Coronary occlusion is total closure of the coronary artery. Coronary thrombosis means a blood clot, or thrombus, has formed in the coronary artery. Myocardial infarction refers to the actual damage or death of heart muscle due to the blockage.

There are many diseases besides heart attacks which affect the heart and blood vessels. They are called cardiovascular diseases. These diseases are often divided into two groups: those which originate inside the heart and those originating outside the heart which affect the heart. In the first group are diseases such as hypertension, congenital heart disease, and rheumatic fever. A heart attack falls in the second group.

MYTH #9: *A large heart attack is more serious than a small heart attack.*

A small heart attack affecting a vital area can be much more dangerous than a large one that spares such portions of the heart.

Doctors consider the location in explaining the prognosis to patients because complications vary according to the affected area. Heart attacks in the front or anterior wall tend to have a higher death rate than those that affect the lower or inferior wall.

Years ago, all heart attacks were considered severe and all were treated alike. Today doctors classify coronary attacks as severe, moderate, or mild. Treatment is tailored to the severity of the attack.

MYTH #10: *Heart attacks occur during particularly stressful times—a family fight, a rough basketball game, shoveling snow.*

Heart attacks can occur any time—under any circumstances. They may strike when a person is having an argument, playing tennis, sitting in a chair, or even sleeping.

Years ago, people believed stress caused heart attacks. Today doctors believe it is just one contributing factor, but an important factor.

The dangerous type of stress is prolonged excessive stress. Two Amsterdam doctors, H. Kits Van Heijeningen and N. Treurnit, believe that almost invariably the period directly preceding a heart attack involves two kinds of stress: trouble at home and trouble at work. In studying thirty men under fifty-six who had heart attacks, they discovered that most were extremely hardworking and had suffered some sort of setback—a loss of income or prestige— in their work. This poor job situation was reinforced by a poor home situation.

MYTH #11: *I will gain weight because I can't be physically active.*

"I went to the hospital at 196 pounds. I came out at 175. Now I'm 176 and going down," one patient recalled.

Immediately after your heart attack, you will probably lose weight. For the first few days in the hospital you may have a liquid diet—broth, fruit juice, and tea. Later, you might be given four or five light meals rather than three large ones.

Most doctors advise heart patients to lose weight because overweight makes the heart do extra work. Overweight people are more prone to high blood pressure. They also get more blood lipid abnormalities that can hasten the development of atherosclerosis.

It is not necessary to be inactive after a heart attack. In fact, it's dangerous. Exercise is important. Since you will probably be eating less and perhaps exercising more, you will probably lose weight.

MYTH #12: *A person who has had a heart attack is never normal again.*

There are some people who seem to derive a kind of pleasure from playing sick and who actually enjoy the sympathy and solicitude of family and friends. The fact is, once a person has recovered from a heart attack there is no cause for sympathy.

A scar on the heart can be no more dangerous than a vaccination scar. While people who have heart attacks are advised to stay under the care of a physician, it should be recognized that there are cases (and there are a great many of them) in which recovery was achieved without medical attention and no future heart attack ever occurred.

Dr. Myron Prinzmetal, a renowned heart specialist, tells the following story of a retired seventy-four-year-old dentist who came to him for treatment:

"He reported that twenty-five years earlier he had been awakened early in the morning with severe pain in the heart region that radiated out to both arms, and at the same time, he felt that he was being suffocated. The pain, he said, lasted for several hours but he thought it was nothing more than acute indigestion and didn't bother to call a doctor. Next day, he went to work. Two years went by, and then one day he suffered a similar set of pains. But again, he didn't even consult a physician and went about his work, standing on his feet all day, practicing dentistry. He continued for years without special treatment until he reached the respectable seventies. Electrocardiograms showed the two old coronary occlusions."

Dr. Prinzmetal points out that this man lived to a ripe old age with no medical attention whatsoever, despite his heart attacks. There are thousands of people like him.

MYTH #13: *A heart attack means you must make drastic changes in your lifestyle.*

Changes in lifestyle are usually not as drastic as you may have anticipated. After a heart attack, most people resume a *normal* active life. Normal is the key.

"I was a junk-food nut. Mallomars—morning, noon, and night. I even kept some in my desk," one patient confessed.

"My day began at seven o'clock. I was at the office by seven-

thirty and didn't get home until ten-thirty—seven days a week
. . . Sundays too," another man commented.

"We're social people. We eat out seven nights a week. I had a
tremendous business lunch and a tremendous dinner every day,"
a young heart victim said.

These lifestyles must be changed, but they were not normal.
Doctors generally recommend that patients stop smoking, lose
weight, and reduce physical and emotional stress in their life. They
may also recommend an exercise program. Some patients are placed
on medications, which must be taken regularly. Other than this,
life basically returns to normal.

MYTH #14: *One heart attack means you'll have another for
sure.*

No one knows whether a person will or will not have a second
heart attack. Compared to people who have had no heart attack,
the risk is increased—but only slightly.

If you have heeded the warning of the first attack and followed the doctor's recommendations about weight, diet, work,
exercise, and rest, your chances of another heart attack may be
markedly decreased. The important thing is to follow competent
medical advice.

MYTH #15: *A second attack is more serious than the first
and a third attack is fatal.*

Second and third attacks can just as well be minor as major.
Indeed, some people have recovered from as many as seven heart
attacks!

MYTH #16: *Skipped heartbeats and palpitations are sure
signs of heart disease.*

Though skipped heartbeats and palpitations may signal heart
disease, they are more commonly symptoms of a healthy heart dis-
turbed temporarily by nervousness, anxiety, or stimulants. Dizziness, trembling, and excessive sighing can sometimes mistakenly
be considered heart "troubles." Again, these may be due to unrelated conditions and have nothing to do with the heart. However,
deciding what is a significant symptom is strictly a medical matter;
self-diagnosis can be dangerous.

MYTH #17: *A diagnosed heart murmur always indicates heart disease.*

Not always. What doctors call a "heart murmur" is actually an alteration in the kind of sound the heart produces as it sends blood through its valves into the blood vessels. Whether or not the murmur indicates heart disease depends on the nature of the sound, where it is most clearly heard, and its relation to the heart's rhythm.

The important murmurs are the ones that develop because of damaged or defective valves. Most other murmurs or noises produced by the heart are harmless. Harmless murmurs are frequently found in children who generally outgrow them.

Most people worry after a heart attack; that is normal and healthy. However, some people and their families become excessively worried. As one man told us, "I feel great but my wife just can't stop worrying about me. If I just sneeze, she amplifies it into something awful."

Half the battle in preventing unnecessary and unhealthy anxiety is understanding. We have begun by dispelling myths. Now let's look at dealing emotionally and physically with the facts.

3. Your Emotional Outlet

A HEART ATTACK is a psychological as well as biological event. Coping with feelings can be even more difficult than taking medicine, restricting diet, or even surgery. Yet a person's psychological attitude toward his disease can be the most important factor in his recovery.

If a person adopts a resigned and fearful attitude, he may indeed become an invalid. However, if his approach is that of someone who has received a shock but is determined to resume life where he left off, he may find his chances for a complete recovery are excellent. From all current research, one message stands out: After a heart attack, people undergo a great deal of psychological stress that *can* be avoided.

Making a psychological adjustment involves understanding a whole mixture of feelings:

1. *You may be depressed.* "I wasn't myself; I began to withdraw," one fifty-year-old man recalled. The courage a person mustered while in the hospital may wear thin by the time he comes home. People may feel lonely. They may be discouraged about changing their lifestyles. They may feel more "down" than they ever have before.
2. *You may be anxious.* Heart attacks bring you close to death. Most people react to the threat of death by becoming anxious. Anxiety occurs during the first few days in the hospital; depression comes later but remains longer.
3. *You may be angry.* "My brother was always angry," a thirty-two-year-old woman said. "If I were to suggest anything, he'd become explosive. He picks on everyone—attacks everyone. It's understandable, but it's still very hard to take."

4. *You may be worried.* "I was extremely worried in the hospital," one salesman recounted. "In fact, I was much more worried about the bills than about the attack. Everyone said 'You need to be there, don't worry about the money,' but I said the hell with that. I wanted to know what it would cost. I was worried that I'd lose my job, that my pay would be cut. I was concerned about how my family would manage."

5. *You may be tense.* For most people, daily life is filled with tension and aggravation. These stresses are intensified by a heart attack. Learning to pace yourself emotionally, to forget bothersome things and go on to something else is one of the most important lessons of a heart attack.

6. *You may fear the future.* When someone is told he definitely had a heart attack, especially a first one, the person is likely to feel a great deal of fear, even if he doesn't show it. He is worried and afraid that any minute his heart will stop altogether.

By examining these and other feelings, you can better understand and handle your emotions. It is very important to recognize that a certain amount of depression, anger, and anxiety are normal and healthy. Moods vary a great deal for several months. When depression, despair, hostility, and withdrawal go on and on, however, it must be recognized as diverging from the normal. Techniques are available to deal with these crisis situations. Knowing what to do and who to contact can significantly help in returning to a normal life.

Depression

"Every patient experiences depression after a heart attack," one New York City cardiologist reported. "It's uniform. I've never seen a patient who did not become depressed."

The degree varies. A person might feel very depressed and cry a lot. When asked why, he may say "I just don't know." On the other hand, some people are unaware they are depressed. They may only be aware of feeling weak, tired, and dependent on others.

Depression often hits hardest when the person goes home, but the veneer may begin to crack in the hospital. Trivial things—a wrong tray—may lead to a temper tantrum. For no reason, an argument may develop with a nurse or orderly. When the doctor says "You're doing great," the patient may privately think "I'm not doing well at all, but he's afraid to tell me."

The person who has heart surgery may experience depression *before* the surgery rather than afterward. One young man who had a triple bypass and was the father of two-year-old twins at the time, explained, "Four or five days before the surgery I was depressed; I had sleepless nights. Finally, I became resigned to my fate, I was cool as ice just before the surgery. I felt like I was going to watch a movie when they wheeled me downstairs. I didn't have depression afterwards. I guess I took care of it in advance."

Depression is due to many factors. It may be caused by unreleased tension and aggression. When aggression is turned inward, depression results. Guilt might also be present. You might feel guilty for somehow causing the heart attack. "If only I had quit that job or stopped smoking," you might say.

Depression is also related to a sense of loss, specifically a loss that affects someone's total future. While the death of a loved one, divorce, or loss of money are obvious losses, a heart attack also causes a sense of permanent loss. It represents the loss of part of your heart, and with it, a loss of a sense of immortality. It is the loss of feeling healthy. If a person's job is affected, there may also be a financial loss.

Depression may be due to role reversals. "I always carried the groceries to the car. My wife doesn't complain, but now she pulls the wagon. I feel perfectly fine. Still, it's a reminder, and it's tough to take," one man said.

Some depressions may be chemically based. When the heart muscle dies, by-products go into the bloodstream. Perhaps the body produces antibodies to these heart substances, and scientists are now wondering whether these chemical changes cause depression.

Whatever the cause, treating depression is essential. Depression may be associated with elevation of lipids (fats and cholesterol) in the bloodstream. High lipid levels are thought to be a major cause of atherosclerosis.

Are You Depressed?

Depressed people generally look depressed. They will have some, but not all, of the following characteristics:

- sad look
- difficulty sleeping and early awakening
- listlessness and disinterest
- inability to concentrate
- expressions of hopelessness or pessimism
- speaking with short verbal responses
- withdrawal (appear to sleep more, want curtains to remain drawn)
- loss of appetite
- uncontrolled crying and easy tearfulness

Some people only look depressed. In fact, they are going through a stage of circumspection in which they are evaluating their problem and trying to figure out the best means of coping with it.

What You Can Do about Depression

A major trauma has been experienced and a certain amount of depression is natural and normal. In fact, some mental health experts view depression as a positive first step toward psychological recovery. They say it represents an acceptance of the current situation and an attempt to come to terms with it.

Regular body exercise can help lift depression. It can use up energies that need to be released and prevent internalization of aggression. Obviously all exercise must be sensibly approached and should be checked by your doctor. Generally, the best way to get started on an exercise program is walking.

Relaxation is important. The first thing a psychiatrist often asks a person is, "What do you do to relax?" Many people, particularly Type A personalities, never relax. (For a full explanation of Type A personality see page 135.) They are workaholics. Television and hobbies are excellent ways to relax. Some people enjoy joining organizations.

It is a big morale booster to wear street clothes during the day. If you plan a nap, change into pajamas, but then back to street clothes. You feel depressed when you look depressed, so it is important to dress and shave each morning.

A helpful tip:

Answer the door when visitors arrive. You will set yourself in an active role from the beginning. Other people will see you that way. Even more importantly, you will see yourself as an active contributing individual.

Anxiety

After a heart attack, most people feel anxious, extremely nervous ("more nervous than I've ever been in my entire life," one patient admitted), and insecure.

Anxiety is an uncomfortable feeling of apprehension which can be either vague or very intense. It is a reaction to a threat to personal security. Anxiety is usually highest in three periods: (1) admission; (2) transfer from the CCU to the regular room ("When you go to the room, you get nervous. You know the nurses are there but they just don't come that fast," a woman who had had two heart attacks explained); (3) before discharge ("I wanted to stay just one more day, even one more minute," one patient said. "And I'll admit when I first got home, I wished I was back").

Anxiety is closely related to inability to anticipate the future. Even the anticipation of an unfavorable outcome is anxiety reducing when it allows the patient to plan and take action to deal with the future.

Not all anxiety is bad. Studies show that patients without anxiety about their condition do not fare well. Anxiety may make people change their unhealthy lifestyle. It may motivate them to comply with instructions concerning diet, exercise, smoking, and stressful work without a sense of loss.

Are You Anxious?

Anxious people are extremely nervous. They have some, but not all, of the following traits:

- excessive talking
- inability to concentrate
- restlessness
- insomnia
- sweating of the palms
- rapid heart beat (tachycardia, doctors call it)

Coping with anxiety is essential, because untreated anxiety leads to depression.

What You Can Do about Anxiety

Anxiety also makes physiological demands on the heart. It can cause complications due to the effects of adrenaline (a catecholamine) mobilization. Catecholamines are activated by stress. Catecholamines increase the work of the heart by increasing heart rate and the force of the contractions. Rigid coronary vessels cannot respond to these increased requirements. Thus, angina, heart failure, and pulmonary edema may result. Therefore, the prevention of anxiety must be a top priority.

Helping around the house diffuses anxiety. "Begin to be useful," Dr. Rubenstein suggests.

"I've been out to business every day of my life and I don't want to start doing housework now," many men reply. If you give it a chance, accomplishing specific tasks can ease mental stress. Drying the dishes, setting the table, mounting old photographs are things that can be undertaken.

A full expression of your emotions is extremely important: "I'm very very scared about returning to work . . . I don't think I can handle it"; "I'm not the man I was"; "I can't do it any more." These fears are very common after a heart attack—they should be honestly aired.

A helpful tip:

Ask questions. Make a list of the things that are worrying you. Call or visit your doctor and discuss them point by point. Have someone else present if possible—a spouse, son, or daughter. This is not so they can talk behind your back but so answers are not forgotten or misconstrued. Take notes; anxiety feeds on the unknown. Being fully informed will dissolve anxiety and worry before they build up.

Denial

Some patients, particularly young people in their thirties and forties, simply deny they had a heart attack. "Well, doctors do make mistakes," is the reasoning. A young man who may have been grappling unsuccessfully with the idea of middle age may reject the whole idea of a heart attack.

Denial usually appears around the second day, and normally will begin dissipating by the third or fourth day. A defense mechanism used to alleviate anxiety by reducing the threat, denial is not only normal, but necessary and healthy. It only becomes a problem when it is prolonged (one or two weeks) and interferes with proper care.

A very common denial pattern is to focus on a very minor physical problem, one that is easier for the person to handle. Dr. Rubenstein gave the following example. "A patient may be very seriously ill. Finally, he will pull through. The next day, he'll smile and say, 'Doc, I feel terrific, but see this little mole over here? Do you think it should be removed?' This happens over and over."

Statements such as "It must be gas"; "It's not possible"; "This couldn't happen to me," show denial.

Denial is serious when it interferes with care. A thirty-two-year-old woman whose twin brother experienced a serious attack commented, "Some people have a heart attack and then take care of themselves. My brother isn't like that. He constantly says 'Don't tell me what to do.' I find if I try to suggest anything, he becomes explosive. He's just not doing anything to take care of himself. He's started to smoke again and I'm afraid drinking is going to be the next step."

What You Can Do about Denial

According to one noted psychiatrist, "The patient may not be deliberately refusing to believe what has happened to him. He simply *can't* believe it."

But he must learn to believe it and adhere to restrictions. One patient in the CCU who refused to obey limitations left the ward without permission to get a newspaper. At the hospital newspaper stand, he had another heart attack. The thirty-two-year-old man described above had a third heart attack only two months later.

A woman who had two heart attacks told us, "I feel okay and I say to myself maybe I can do a little more, but no dice. The minute I do more, I feel it. I get the pressure, and I have to open my mouth for breathing. I have to stop."

"You have to respect the disease," another victim commented. Although most cardiac conditions are amenable to therapy, relatively few are completely curable. The vast majority of cardiac patients have to live with their disease permanently. Doctors can diagnose and prescribe. The lifestyle is entirely up to the patient. It is difficult but important to impress these factors on heart patients who tend to deny their disease.

Overdependency

Some men, particularly older men, may revert to childlike dependence on their family. At first all patients are very dependent. "When they arrive in the CCU, they are very, very passive and dependent," said Marilyn Citron, head CCU nurse at Beth Israel Hospital in New York City.

All hospitalized patients undergo regression, and this is especially true of heart patients. From the beginning, they are treated like children. They are fed, washed, and helped with all bodily functions. Moving from extreme dependence into independence after discharge is not an easy transition, but excessive dependence can cause a person to become a cardiac cripple.

Sometimes extreme dependency is based on subconscious motivation. Some people may have long been looking for just such an excuse to avoid the responsibilities of life. They see the heart attack as an "out," an excuse to finally retire. Although they may be perfectly capable of returning to work, they refuse to do so. They may speak constantly about their terrible brush with death and feelings of impending doom.

What You Can Do about Overdependence

First and foremost, it is important for family and associates to understand that psychological rather than physical factors are causing this behavior. With time, reassurance, and persuasion, the person may eventually be led back to a productive life.

Independence can be encouraged by giving a person a share in decisions about his own care. Have him select his bath time, choose his menus, plan his outdoor strolls. Ask him things he knows the answer to; this enhances feelings of competence.

Usually overdependence lessens with time. Rarely, people are unable to overcome excessive dependency. In such cases, professional counseling is advisable.

Minor Discomforts and Fears of Another Attack

After going home, a person may notice minor chest aches that are often due to small irritations of the rib joints and chest muscles.

The doctor may have repeatedly asked you if you have any chest pain or shortness of breath, so you are watching for it. When people are in normal health, they have minor aches and pains. However, every little pain becomes alarming after a heart attack. Some people must take one or two deep breaths periodically. This usually is caused by anxiety and not by heart problems.

What You Can Do about Minor Discomforts and Fears
of Another Attack

To help you sort out the important from the unimportant pains, you should be aware that pain from the heart (angina or another heart attack) will usually recur in the same location. It will also, in general, have the same feeling as the pain suffered in the heart attack. Taking nitroglycerin will also help you differentiate heart pain from other body discomfort. In general, pain originating in the heart will be relieved by nitroglycerin within one or two minutes, whereas other pain will be unaffected by nitroglycerin.

Some people are alarmed by short-lasting stabbing pains in the heart area which are severe enough to inhibit them from taking a deep breath. Such discomfort lasts only a few seconds, at most a minute, and is unrelated to physical exertion. It often hits while sitting and often improves with forced exhaling. This is usually *not* heart trouble. Most frequently, nervous eating and constant swallowing of excess air are the cause.

Significant shortness of breath usually occurs when a person is walking or climbing stairs rather than sitting. It is likely to be accompanied by a fast pulse. A person lying flat on his back and complaining of shortness of breath usually does not have a serious problem either; if he did, he would sit up or walk around to try to find some relief.

Deciding what is or is not a significant symptom is *not* the layman's job. A physician should definitely be consulted. Some people feel embarrassed about going to a doctor, fearing there is nothing wrong. Another group of people tend to minimize all symptoms fearing the doctor *will* find something wrong. Both attitudes are dangerous.

Since the greatest risk of death occurs during the first few hours of a heart attack, it is obvious that a doctor should be consulted promptly for any chest pain or shortness of breath.

Fatigue

Fatigue is the most common complaint after hospital discharge. All the patients we interviewed complained about feeling exhausted. A thirty-nine-year-old teacher who suffered an uncomplicated heart attack was a typical example. He said, "I felt great in the hospital. No matter what anyone told me I pictured myself breaking records getting back to work. The first week home I could hardly walk the length of the house without feeling exhausted. I felt like a cooked goose, like I was done for. It took another two weeks before I started to feel better."

Fatigue may be due to depression, but most likely, it is just a normal part of the recovery. However, it may indicate a further cardiac problem.

What You Can Do about Fatigue

After a heart attack, people feel unbelievably weak and tired. They should be prepared for this. Weakness is not a sign of complication. It does not mean that a heart condition is getting worse or that a person will always feel like this. Rather, it is an expected part of the recovery.

Sometimes, however, fatigue can be significant. If a person has a hard day, sleeps poorly, and feels completely exhausted and washed out the next day, he should speak to his doctor. If a person feels tired in the midst of an activity, he should stop immediately and rest until he feels normal again. The idea is to stop *before* feeling tired.

If someone feels "just exhausted" all the time, he should speak with his doctor. Only a physician can accurately evaluate the meaning of such fatigue.

Nightmares

"I had such terrible nightmares, I finally called my doctor," one successful fifty-four-year-old business executive told us. "When I was a little boy about nine or ten we had a tractor. One day I was playing around, backing up the tractor. I didn't see an old man behind me and I knocked him over. I got a very bad scolding from my mother. In my dream, I killed the man. I haven't thought about that incident in forty-five years."

What You Can Do about Nightmares

Drugs taken after a heart attack can cause nightmares. Inderal, a commonly used pill for controlling angina and hypertension, can cause nightmares.

Sleeping pills can cause nightmares after they are discontinued. It is important to know that when you stop taking sleeping pills you get a "rebound effect." This means you will spend 40 to 50 percent of the night dreaming. These dreams often have a nightmarish quality.

Bad dreams of smothering or drowning may also be signs of psychological stress. Some people who are extremely anxious grind their teeth during their sleep.

Anger and Hostility

Hostility is a double problem. The patient might have simmering rage, and his wife or partner might also feel angry and put-upon. Marriages frequently break up due to the anger and hostility after a heart attack. Therefore, treating hostility is a top priority.

"My wife resented the fact that I was sick," a forty-year-old man told us. "She made me feel like I had some nerve having a heart attack and needing surgery. 'What the hell do you want me to do?' I'd say. It was tough. But we both did a little growing."

What You Can Do about Anger and Hostility

To defuse hostility, one must get to the root of it. Was there hostility before the heart attack? Was the person passive-aggressive for years? Is the heart attack really to blame? These are important questions. If other matters seem to be at the root of the trouble, discussing the situation with a cardiologist would be helpful.

It is normal for both parties to feel angry. Within certain limits this anger should be expressed. Internalized anger could cause depression. Dr. Howard A. Wishnie stated in the JAMA article "Psychological Hazards of Convalescence Following Myocardial Infarction," "Wives should be cautioned against totally suppressing appropriate annoyance or anger as these responses may emerge in the guise of zealous overprotection, among others, and cause more disruption than in the original form."

Anger can be dissipated without continual arguments. Anna Burton, a leading New Jersey psychoanalyst suggests the following anger-alleviating methods:

1. Have a "talking time" each day. After breakfast, before dinner, while driving to the grocery store are good informal times. This dissipates anger before it builds.
2. Have visitors. Dr. Burton suggests just one every day to avoid fatigue. But again, she emphasizes this should be every day, or every other day, to prevent the build-up of hostility.
3. Make special plans six months in advance. This takes the mind off current pressures.
4. Go outdoors. A person who has been sick may experience nature with new eyes. Pleasant sensations have an easing mental effect.

Boredom

Boredom is a common complaint because of enforced inactivity and restrictions immediately after a heart attack.

What You Can Do about Boredom

Boredom is, in some ways, a good sign. It shows the person is recovering. Dr. Joseph S. Alpert, in *The Heart Attack Handbook* suggests, "Try to choose activities that are varied and relaxing, and plan a number of different ones for each day. Reading and handicrafts are frequently good cures for boredom."

"I read anything and everything on heart disease," several people told us. They found this passed the time, and also gave them a better understanding of their problem.

A helpful tip:

While in the hospital, go to occupational therapy. There is no additional charge and it can provide some interesting new interests and hobbies.

Fear of Death

Of all the fears after a heart attack, two predominate: fear of death and fear of living with impending death. People are more afraid of having something wrong with their heart than any other organ. To many, heart disease means "dropping dead." How these fears are handled can greatly affect a person's mental and physical recovery. It is important that people are not continually anxious. This can increase the chances of another attack.

"Most healthy people can't conceptualize death," Dr. Rubenstein explained. "There is a healthy denial pattern. People don't really come to grips with their own mortality until they are ill or threatened."

"After my bypass surgery, I did have a feeling of sadness," one forty-six-year-old social worker explained. "Before that, I was fat, dumb, and happy. I thought I could do anything under the sun, and I did. I smoked, I drank, and I partied. After the operation I felt vulnerable. My horse had left the barn, and I wished he were back."

Everyone is frightened by a heart attack. Some express fear, but most don't explicitly say, "I think I'm going to die." However, reassurance is important for everyone.

What You Can Do about Fear of Death

"We are not God and today patients know it," a young cardiologist explained. "I don't really know if someone will or will not die. It's very hard to predict with heart attacks. I tell them I will do everything humanly possible to pull them through. Then I work like hell. I'll be there and they know it. It's comforting."

For more reassurance, the American Red Cross and various

hospitals offer classes in the techniques of cardiopulmonary resuscitation (CPR). It makes people feel better knowing that, if
necessary, they can save someone's life.

Dealing with Your Feelings

No one is perfect before or after a heart attack. Psychological
problems may exist from childhood.

By and large, people react to illness according to long-estab-
lished personality patterns. As one wife admitted, "He was always
selfish, even before his heart attack. We used to call him a bear.
Now we call him a brute."

All patients experience emotional problems after a heart attack. As Dr. Theodore Cooper, Dean of Cornell University Medical
College pointed out, "You can't deal with stress by withdrawing from
your life situation and your community and trying to escape into
isolation. All that amounts to is the substitution of one form of
stress for another. You may think it is the easiest way out, but you
do not solve problems by making believe they aren't there—by cop-
ping out."

Many ways to deal with feelings have already been suggested.
If do-it-yourself methods do not work, professional assistance should
be sought. Your family doctor might refer you to a psychiatrist or a
psychologist for individual or group therapy; or he may recommend
drugs.

Having Therapy

Psychiatric help is nothing shameful. One leading New York
City medical center requires *all* heart attack patients to speak with
a psychiatrist before discharge.

Therapy does not have to be long-term. It may take just a few
sessions or one or two months. Regardless, it is best to deal with a
psychiatrist or psychologist experienced in the interrelationship between psychological problems and physical disease.

"I've never had a patient who asked to speak to a therapist,"
said Marilyn Citron, head nurse of the Coronary Care Unit at Beth

Israel Hospital in New York City. However, the nurses or doctors may suggest counseling. Ms. Citron explains, "If the denial pattern is very strong—you know the patient who is ready to have the phone hooked up, papers brought in, and conduct business as usual here in the CCU—we will seek a consultation." Excessive depression, over-dependency, and anxiety can also be helped by counseling.

Group therapy for wives and patients, alone and/or together, is offered by many hospitals and cardiac clubs. Group therapy shows a person the universality of many of his worries and anxieties. It also provides peer support in dealing with common but often unex-pressed feelings such as anger, loss of privacy, and loss of dignity.

Though, ideally, people should discuss these feelings with fam-ily, friends, nurses, and physicians, in reality these opportunities are limited. It is easier to talk with others who share these problems.

While all patients would benefit from some counseling, few re-quire long-term therapy. One cardiologist estimated one patient in twenty, roughly 5 percent, require such psychiatric help.

"I find patients who need long-term psychiatric help have long-standing problems in their psychological makeup," Dr. Rubenstein explains. "The heart attack was just enough to push them over. It may have been the catalyst, but the problems were present for years."

After a heart attack, some people complain continuously. It is tempting to disregard this as "needless bitching" or admonish some-one for "acting like a child." But it is important to remember that frustration affects blood lipid levels which, in turn, affect the heart. People with abnormally high expectations of personal care and at-tention who are prone to frustration and anger when their demands aren't met might need special counseling.

What You Should Know about Mood-Changing Drugs

After a heart attack, doctors routinely give tranquilizers and sleeping pills. Some patients do not like to take these drugs because they are afraid of addiction; others see them as a sign of weakness. When used following a heart attack, these pills are rarely, if ever, addictive. In an event as traumatic as a heart attack, it is not a sign of weakness but an important therapy.

Antidepressant drugs are *not* routinely given. However, in cases of moderate to severe depression, they may be prescribed.

Tranquilizers. Tranquilizers are antianxiety pills that calm the nerves, sooth anxieties, and relax a person. The most commonly prescribed are Valium and Librium. Tranquilizers do not treat depression. In fact, as a side effect, tranquilizers can make some people cry more easily, feel depressed, and get extremely angry.

Taken over a long period of time, some tranquilizers and antidepressants can produce changes in the electrocardiogram without actually damaging the heart. These changes usually go away if the drug is stopped. No tranquilizers should ever be taken unless a doctor is consulted. Some of these pills can interfere with the actions of high-blood-pressure pills.

Sleeping Pills. The most commonly prescribed sleeping pill is Dalmane, because it does not contain barbiturates. Some people consider taking nonprescription sleeping pills. The most common are Dromin, Nytol, Sleep-Eze, and Sominex. Their main sedative ingredient is an antihistamine drug that is promoted as a sleeping pill because of the drowsiness it produces. Absolutely no sleeping pills should be taken, no matter how seemingly harmless, without consulting a physician.

Antidepressant Pills. If depression is moderate to severe (you can feel very low and still have "mild" depression) antidepressant drugs may be prescribed. There are several different types of antidepressants but the most common are amitriptyline (Elavil) and impiramine (Tofranil). For antidepressant drugs to be effective, full doses must be taken for three to six months.

There have been cases of death with some antidepressants in heart patients. Therefore, they should be taken only under the close supervision of a physician.

A New Look at Life

All emotions after a heart attack are not negative ones. Most people feel immensely grateful and happy to be alive.

Unquestionably, they are the lucky ones. Over a million people suffer heart attacks each year, half die before ever reaching the hospital.

A middle-aged man, after matter-of-factly discussing his illness and recovery, began to cry, saying, "I never knew anyone cared about me. I just never knew." A young patient thoughtfully remarked, "I found out just how tenuous life can be and I really do enjoy every day with a new sense of reality."

4. What Your Family Is Feeling

THE EXPERIENCE a family encounters when heart attack strikes is a harrowing one; the emotional scars can last for years. The moving account of Jane Feldman, a thirty-four-year-old interior designer is perhaps typical.

"My father was a very strong figure. I was afraid of him, but if there was any major problem, I knew he would know what to do. He was never sick a day in his life. I was totally protected.

"He liked girls and I was a typical teenager—popular, blond, and bubbly. My brother was gentle—not a typical boy—and father always favored me. He thought women should be pretty and lead protected lives.

"All of a sudden, at age forty-two, he had a heart attack. I came home at the end of my sophomore year of college and overnight everything changed. I found it totally devastating. Before he had been the strong one—he worked fourteen hours a day, played three sets of tennis at a time. Now he couldn't even carry a suitcase. All of a sudden, I couldn't go home to the father I had known and I was positively terrified.

"He would get upset when you tried to talk about it. Mother would say, 'Don't upset your father.' So we just didn't talk—we just didn't mention it. I tuned out more and more, and stayed away from home so I wouldn't have to deal with it.

"I resented him for getting sick. And I was scared. Sometimes he'd get emotional and cry. The first time I saw it, I was devastated. I was scared stiff.

"I never realized all of this until after he died. He was at a convention in Florida. My mother called at 4:30 A.M. I became hysterical for thirty seconds, then I gained perfect control. I washed my hair, dressed, and went to the airport. When I got to Florida, I tried to sleep, but my whole body ached. The pain in my body was un-believable. Then in the year after he died, all of this anger came out at my mother. It was because of the total suppression for all those years.

"I'm not the type who admits I'm scared so I covered up in other ways. I just stayed away. My mother thought I just wasn't interested, so she began to resent me, and made me feel guilty. Why didn't I visit the hospital more? Why didn't I come home more?

"I think if we had talked about it, things would have been bet-ter. At the hospital, there should have been a program for families —mothers and children. You can't leave children out. If they know what to expect, if they are allowed to talk, things would be better. But when the person is discharged, everyone flounders. You try to cope, but sometimes you have to be shown the right way."

A very attractive fifty-year-old woman gave us this account of her husband's recent heart attack.

"There are so many emotions—so many hates, so many loves, so much anger. More than anything, you feel terribly inadequate. There is so little you can do for someone you love. It's all dependent on others and God and, unfortunately, I'm not a great believer in the deity. I'm from the school where you depend on yourself. All of a sudden you are totally dependent on strangers. Often you get the feeling they couldn't care less. You wait hours for a lousy pillow, and then they'll send an orderly. If you have pain, you can wait hours for relief. I found it appalling.

"We never had much contact with doctors and nurses before. Thank God, we're a healthy family. We never think about illnesses. I found that doctors don't talk to wives. If they talk at all, they talk down or they talk doctorese. Or they talk with one foot out the door.

"When they do talk, it is so hard to listen. You want to push it away. They are talking to you but you don't want to hear bad news. You want them to tell you everything will be all right. You listen hard, but emotions take over so completely. You are so upset, you just don't hear.

"My husband is an easy man, but he was a terribly difficult patient. He refused to believe he had a heart attack. One of the doc-tors had to come in and yell at him and say 'Look here, you really did have a heart attack.' He wanted out of the hospital. When the TV broke, he screamed and wanted to climb on the ceiling to fix it. He screamed at everybody—and he screamed at me. He'd say 'Get out. Don't visit. Don't bother coming.' I had very mixed emotions. I was teary. I felt sorry for myself. And I was ashamed of him. After he got out of the CCU, things got better. But the initial period was extremely tough.

"I'm not a talker—I kept everything inside. The only one I could really talk with is my sister. Talking with my sister settled me down. I talked with her on the phone. When she was there, I relaxed. I wasn't as relaxed with my children (they are thirty and twenty-five) as I was with my sister. In fact, sometimes I must admit I resented them. They were greatly concerned but they were busy doing their own thing, living their own lives. I felt they came when it was convenient for them.

"When he came home, I felt great joy but also great fear. I had the feeling that if I did something wrong, it would happen again. I didn't want to make an invalid out of my husband. You shouldn't constantly ask 'How are you feeling?' but I just couldn't stop myself. I am constantly thinking heart attack. I know all the worrying in the world doesn't change anything, but you don't have an 'off' button to push. Although I know all the right things to say, it's hard to change. I hear myself saying 'How do you feel?' and I know I should stop. I hate myself for doing it, but it comes out.

"We were good sex partners. He says it's even better now, but I have great fears. The doctor said we could have relations, but I find that I am petrified. Sometimes the fear subsides a bit but it never completely goes away. I don't think you ever get over it.

"For me, I'm still waking up in the middle of the night to see that he's breathing. If he gets up to go to the bathroom, I ask 'How do you feel?' or 'What's the matter?'

"This year we went on a vacation with friends. I wanted to have people with us because we were so far away from the doctor. When he went swimming I was nervous as can be—I had to walk away. I was constantly thinking what if he had a heart attack out there. I'm not such a good swimmer. How would we ever reach him?

"I think his heart attack brought us closer. In fact, I know it has. We both feel we came so close to losing each other. We've been married thirty-six years. And, you know, your spouse is always just there. Suddenly you find it's all so fragile . . . all hanging by a thread. You are immensely grateful. You just don't take each other for granted any more. You appreciate in a new and deeper sense."

While difficulties are the rule, one medical secretary gave us this account of her husband's attack.

"Dennis had his heart attack in 1973. He was forty-nine and had been diabetic since he was twenty-two. Now he noticed he had the first and third leading causes of death. But he sort of kids about it. He doesn't act frightened, that's why I'm not frightened. He never thinks of himself as a sick man, so it rubs off on me. Neither of us have a frightened feeling.

"It happened on the street. They brought him right to the hospital, and within one hour he was in the Coronary Care Unit. He recovered uneventfully. Then he stayed home for three months. I found myself waking up at night listening to him breathe. I'm still overly concerned. If he gets tired, I immediately ask why is he tired.

"When I was first called and met him at the emergency room, I couldn't believe it. I was very, very afraid he would die. I have a nervous stomach, so immediately I was in the bathroom.

"The doctor told me every twelve hours were important. So when seventy-two hours passed, I started to live with the fact that although he had a heart attack, he'd get better. When he recovered, I felt he was totally recovered. I didn't think he should be shielded from anything. He's my husband; he must be part of everything. We had the normal confrontations with the kids. We had our fights.

"I thought, at the beginning, my life would be preoccupied with Dennis's heart attack, but it really hasn't been. We try to be health-minded. He walks to and from work each day. Basically, our life is like it always was."

Certainly there are no easy answers. People who have suffered heart attacks can be difficult to live with. The first week home can be particularly trying.

Three cardinal rules may help ease tensions:

RULE #1: *Talk, talk talk.*

Acknowledging honest feelings and openly discussing them makes a vast difference.

"My husband keeps everything inside," many women say. This is not unusual. But sharing on a feeling level after a heart attack is essential.

"I was afraid to talk about it. I thought it would remind him. I was afraid I'd just upset him and make matters worse," one wife admitted. Actually, talking is comforting. It's keeping things to yourself that brings the problems.

RULE #2: *Expect difficulties.*

Many people feel that illness unifies families. In reality, it often tears close families apart.

"Even under the best of conditions, a wife should expect difficulties," a leading psychiatrist told us. "Husbands and wives are both going to be angry. They will both feel overburdened. They will both be under stress. Tensions result; they are inevitable."

A heart attack victim may be unnaturally preoccupied with himself. He may feel he should be catered to constantly. Family members may be afraid to refuse any request out of fear of causing another attack. In some cases, they may feel guilty about causing the heart attack in the first place.

On the other hand, wives may be over-solicitous. This can be immensely annoying. "I wish my wife would get off my back," many men complain. "Leave me alone," they may say brusquely and then withdraw. One wife admitted, "Every night after dinner, my husband shut the bedroom door and watched TV. He refused to talk."

A young girl recalls, "I think carrying the luggage was the worst part. It sounds like a trivial thing but it would get my father furious. He'd have outbursts. At the end, he was just resigned. The outbursts were easier than the resignation."

RULE #3: *Realize things do get better.*

Time is probably the biggest help. When the person returns to work, pressures ease. As soon as he or she sees life is not as bad as anticipated, things usually *do* get back to normal.

How the Wife Feels

Overwhelmed. Exhausted. Depressed. Beside myself. Angry. These feelings were expressed by many wives.

"The wife is frequently in a 'no-win' situation," Dr. Rubenstein explained. "She is put in a very difficult spot. The responsibility for the diet is placed on the wife. She wants to help her husband and serve the right food, but he may make her the 'whipping boy' because he doesn't want to follow the diet. He may be nasty at the table and blame her. No matter which way she turns, she's wrong."

Wives usually experience depression after their husband's heart attacks. Their anxiety, stress, and fear of loss take a heavy toll. When these emotions have nowhere to go but inward, depression results. This is normal. Nevertheless, it is painful and difficult to cope with. Indeed, a wife's burden is often the most difficult.

Yet there is, perhaps, a silver lining. Over and over, men we spoke with echoed a deeply moving appreciation for their wives' emotional support. "You asked me what pulled me through, two words 'my wife,' " a fifty-three-year-old photographer who suffered three heart attacks told us. "She was extremely supportive in every way. She was concerned. She's a companion—we like being alone together. We are satisfied with each other's company. She was by far the most important thing in my recovery."

Of course, a heart attack cannot turn a bad marriage into a good one. But many people told us that, eventually, they found their marriage had been strengthened. "Before, my wife would give me the silent treatment," one man who had two attacks and whose wife also had two attacks explained. "Now we don't have time to waste in fighting. Life is too precious to waste on nonsense. Of course we still argue. But the arguments don't last like they did before."

Playing Mother Hen

"Don't baby me! The one thing I don't need is another mother," one young man who recently suffered a serious attack angrily shouted at his young wife. Most wives do tend to overprotect their husbands; many admit lying awake at night listening to their husband's every breath. This overprotection is resented by the men. The following example is typical:

A man who recently had a heart attack and a friend were discussing medicines. The man rose to get his pills from a nearby table. His wife, who was seated across the room, jumped to her feet exclaiming, "Wait now, dear, let me get that for you." The man's response was to bolt angrily from his chair and glare furiously at his wife.

Clearly, the emotional upset of this incident far exceeded any physical problem. Aggressive overprotection sometimes reflects suppressed anger. Whatever the motivation, it can cause serious conflicts, even in stable marriages, and should be stringently avoided.

When to Back Off

"A wife must know when to back off," Dr. Rubenstein advises. "If he is constantly annoyed about the diet, she should not keep after him. It's best to compromise. Let him have his favorite foods for a day or two and then try to ease back into it."

How much to back off is a sensitive dilemma. For example, one man had a mother-in-law whom he always disliked. Naturally, she wanted to come and visit after his illness. The wife was put in an awkward position: Should she ban her mother or tell her husband he was being unreasonable? In this case, Dr. Rubenstein suggested, it is probably best to give in to the husband temporarily.

"Could you get the _____ for me, honey?" is another common problem. In dwelling on themselves, some men make their wives slaves. When should the wife say "Enough! Get it yourself"? Dr. Rubenstein suggests that a wife cannot and should not continually wait on her husband. Most wives told us "I didn't have a minute to myself from the second he got sick." This breeds anger, which, in turn, leads to trouble. So the wife must be open, and assure her husband he can do some things for himself.

Despite all of this, wives are told to be cheerful. Everyone knows how difficult this is, but it is important advice. People who are ill are extremely attuned to the mood of others. As a sixty-year-old businessman said, "My wife always smiled; she was always cheerful. We've been married going on thirty-four years. I know her ways: She can hide very little. I know she was scared, but I was glad she didn't show it. She acted 'up' and it helped . . . it really helped a lot."

Some Practical Pointers

Illness complicates life. Here are some practical ways to ease the burden:

1. Go out to eat. It is not necessary to always cook at home to follow new dietary rules. "I was amazed to learn that you can tell restaurants exactly how you'd like the food cooked and they'll do it with no fuss or extra charge," one woman told us. "When I go out, I always order the same—fish, lots of salad, no dressing," a young heart victim explained.
2. When shopping, get a salesperson. Going through clothing racks can be exhausting. A woman, age fifty, who had three heart attacks said, "I went to my favorite store and found a helpful saleswoman. I give her all my business. She understands me, my taste, and even my medical problems. She goes through the racks and picks out some selections for me. Boy, does it make things easier."
3. Find one friend. "I think if you can find just one person to confide in, you'll be okay," the wife of a heart patient told us. Rather than "open up" to everyone, try to confide in just one close friend or relative.
4. See a doctor regularly. Illness shows us the importance of having a regular family physician. One wife told us, "When my husband got the pains, I didn't know who to call. I called my friend who is a nurse and she took us over to the hospital. Now I know the importance of having a regular doctor. My kids haven't seen anyone since they stopped going to the pediatrician. Now I'm insisting."
5. Have things delivered. "I was always pushing that cart and it was just murder," one woman said. By ordering in large quantities, you can make use of delivery services at almost no extra cost.

How the Children Feel

Children are deeply affected by heart attacks. As one twelve-year-old put it, "I was scared at first. Every time Dad mentioned a pain, I went looking through the encyclopedia. When they finally told me it was a heart attack, I wasn't surprised. In fact, it was better then, 'cause we all started to work together."

Feelings of guilt may occur. Selma, a young day-care administrator, told us, "I felt guilty because I had a lot of hostility towards my father. Because we never got along, I had mixed feelings when he got sick. He needed someone to take care of him when he got home. I'm the oldest and I felt it was my responsibility to be there but I didn't want to and I didn't. Even though he's much better now, I still feel guilty."

The most common error in dealing with children is overprotection. "We tried to protect our kids too much and we shouldn't have," one man who suffered a serious attack at age thirty-eight explained. "I think the kids should be included as much as possible. We didn't want to scare them. The truth is, they were scared anyway. When you try to hide things from them, I think fear turns to resentment in some way."

What the Children Can Do

Depending on their age, children can ease the heart attack experience in different ways. A twenty-seven-year-old son took over his father's complex import-export business. He had already worked in the business for two years so the transition was a natural one. His father told us, "The most important thing was I could really relax; I knew the business was in very good hands. He solved problems—I must admit—better than I could have. Of course he never told me he had any problems."

"Dad always wanted to know what was going on," the son added. "I always kept him posted but I told him only the good news. I filtered the rest."

Regardless of age, the important thing is helping. A young boy whose father had a very serious attack advised: "The main thing is to do what is necessary at the time and forget everything else."

The following suggestions were made by children of heart attack victims:

1. Help with the housework. "There was a lot to be done, so we did our best to keep the house organized," a ten-year-old said. "We vacuumed, dusted, and did the laundry."
2. Climb stairs. "After Dad came home he was real tired, so I'd run downstairs if he wanted something," one young boy told us.
3. Keep Dad involved. "I tried to tell him things I was doing in school. Even though he couldn't go to the school play, I told him my entire part. Mom told me to and I think he liked it," a third-grader said.
4. Mow the lawn.
5. Bring fresh fruit to the hospital. "I brought Dad some fresh fruit—all nicely peeled and cut, and he really loved it," a young woman told us.
6. Take out garbage.
7. Do food shopping: Take the groceries home.
8. Take Mom out to dinner. A young man said "My girl friend and I took Mom out for dinner every night after the hospital. It was a pleasant way to end the day, and it kept her from sitting around alone and thinking."
9. Take something to the nurses. "I brought candy for the nurses. Dad felt they were doing so much for him; he wanted to do something for them. It made him happy," a daughter said.
10. Be there. "I think it was helpful that I was there," a twenty-one-year-old son commented. "I helped make things go smoothly and I know Mom appreciated it."

Children Have Hearts Too

After a heart attack, children worry about their parents. But parents worry about their children too. They are concerned that their children may inherit the tendency for heart disease. They wonder if somehow this can be prevented.

Doctors usually advise parents to educate their children about risk factors and the need for reducing them. If one parent had a heart attack at a very early age, many doctors consider it advisable to have the pediatrician run tests for high blood fat levels. If this test shows high levels, dietary changes may be recommended. For high school students, doctors suggest a thorough medical examination at some point before graduation. This should include blood pressure tests as well as tests to determine the levels of cholesterol, triglycerides, uric acid, and blood sugar.

Without question, the best thing parents can do for their children is set a good example. If you smoke, you should stop. Your own example is more significant than all the lectures in the world. Eating a good diet, drinking in moderation, and exercising regularly are all learned by example more than any other way.

Learning to live a healthy life is prudent. However, at no time should concern about heart disease become an obsession—for the parents or children themselves.

A warning:

Some physicians believe that a cholesterol test is not always reliable in an infant. It is also possible that a low-cholesterol diet might interfere with early brain development for which cholesterol is necessary.

Guidelines for How to Act

Families are deeply concerned and frightened by a heart attack. Although it throws their entire life into disarray, it is important to act calmly. The worst thing for a person after an attack is extra worry. The family's job is to provide reassurance. To do this, family members should:

1. *Act optimistic*—even if you don't feel it. It is important not to let fears and concerns show. Optimistic patients do best. If possible, ask the boss to call or visit. This will provide financial reassurance.
2. *Act cheerful*—even if you are overburdened. Sickness brings financial pressures. The hospital room is not the place to bring

up unpaid bills, problems with the children, or household worries. You must put on a strong act.

3. *Act sympathetic*—but not smothering. Though sick, the person is still an adult and should be respected and treated as such.

Once home from the hospital, it may be difficult to follow doctor's orders. As Dr. Marshall Franklin, author of *The Heart Attack Handbook,* put it, "Even the most disciplined patient will grow lax sometimes. If he is feeling well, he is apt to cheat a bit at first, later a little more, especially if there are no repercussions. It's human nature."

Jacqueline Dunbar, coordinator of recruitment and adherence for a coronary prevention program sponsored by the National Heart, Lung and Blood Institute reported that "between 20 and 80 percent of all patients fail to comply with medical advice." She found that "the most notorious among the offenders are asymptomatic individuals assigned to long-term preventive regimes." For success with this problem, Ms. Dunbar has suggested these do's and don'ts:

Do
· Hold down the number of changes to be made.
· Stick with the same health-care team.
· Keep regimes simple.

DON'T
· Continually coax.
· Give "If you don't . . ." warnings.

For more specific guidelines, it is important to understand the person's personality. Different personality types have different emotional needs and different modes of expressing these needs at a time of crisis. A brief description of these personality types and how-to-act suggestions follow.

The Obsessive-Compulsive Personality

Personality Traits. This type of person deals with stress by attempting to structure the situation, place it in order, and systematize it. He is a thinker, questioner, and doubter. By converting the problem into an intellectual one, he turns the situation into something understandable, thus manageable. He removes the awesomeness and mystery.

How to Act. This type of person is reaching out for control, order, and meaning. He will be very uncomfortable with vagueness, indecision, and lack of information. He should be given massive amounts of information so he can understand his illness and the prescribed treatment. It is best for the family to make certain the doctor gives full and explicit information to the patient himself, not just the spouse or children. If the person has more questions, encourage him to speak to the doctor, nurse, or social worker. In providing information, avoid emotionally charged words such as "death" and "heart attack."

The Repressive Personality

Personality Traits. This person is almost opposite to the obsessive compulsive. He may be just as intelligent but in time of stress he prefers to put troublesome things out of his mind, and he wants others to do the same. When something does get his attention, his thoughts are not sharp. Dramatic and over-reactive, emotional outbursts may result.

How to Act. The repressive person does not want to be bothered with detail. He is most comfortable when family members are firm and parental. They should reflect utmost confidence in the professional care he is receiving; the repressive type cannot tolerate doubt.

The Dependent Personality

Personality Traits. Many people deal with crisis by turning fully to an authority in whom they have a great deal of faith. They are aware a crisis exists and they are aware of their own inability to deal with it. There is almost a childlike belief that the health professional is all-wise and all-powerful so no harm is possible.

How to Act. While it is important to wean a person from excessive dependency, some dependence immediately after an attack is beneficial. It enables the person to rest and be properly cared for. However, excessive dependency must not be permitted to continue. Dependency is addictive. Soon the person will not want to leave the hospital. He'll insist on being taken care of long after it is necessary. This type of person must be encouraged to do things for himself—bathing, dressing, and eating. Perhaps the most important thing for the dependent person is constant reassurance. If the family is calm and confident, anxiety will be assuaged. Stability, calmness, and confidence are keys in handling the dependent-type person.

Hyper-Independent Personality

Personality Traits. Often a person who is really very frightened or perhaps ashamed of being very dependent will act in a totally independent manner. He may angrily cast off any attempts to help him. Such a person is trying to show he is not scared; he is not helpless; he is not a child. Because the heart attack situation is one of helplessness, fear, and childlike dependency, this situation is sensitive.

How to Act. Dr. Max Needleman of the Department of Psychiatry at Beth Israel Hospital in New York City advises, "With such a person you must bargain. If you fight him completely, it will create more damage than good. You can't be inflexible because you just won't win."

It is best to allow this type of person to participate in his own care, wherever possible. For instance, ask him if he wants the lights on or off, the shade up or down. At all opportunities, no matter how minor, involve him.

Paranoid Personality

Personality Traits. Some people who have had many difficulties, have been hurt, or have faced many stresses may be basically angry and bitter. A heart attack only increases the anger.

Psychiatrists tell us that hostility is an unconscious attempt to anger others. The nicer and more seductive the person, the greater the threat of liking him and being hurt again, so the greater the antagonism.

How to Act. It is important to let these people express their hostility. However, the family's response should be neither hostile nor overly sweet but neutral. It is important to remember that fear and hurt are motivating this behavior.

Depressive Personality

Personality Traits. Many people respond to a heart attack with overwhelming depression. Feelings of anguish, despair, hopelessness, and even intense guilt and self-disgust may cause them to express the wish that they had never been born or do not want to go on living.

This is especially true of conscientious people. When these people get into difficulty, they tend to blame themselves for their problems, they feel if only they had acted differently, everything would have been all right. Their heart attacks seem to be just one more example of something they did wrong and of not being able to do anything right. They feel they have failed. This may be intensified if they are no longer the breadwinner.

How to Act. For people of this type, it is best to verbally acknowledge their depression. "Gee, you really look down," you might say to let him know you are aware of his emotional turmoil. Positive remarks about progress and possible future plans are also helpful. It is important to be cheerful; don't cry along with the person.

Reinforce competence. This lessens feelings of helplessness. Make him the decision-maker, wherever possible. For example, even in the simple matter of a bath, ask him when he would like it. Encourage him to select his daily menu and consult him on household decisions.

Anna Burton, a leading psychiatrist and psychoanalyst remarked, "A wife should make her husband feel as important and capable as possible. She might ask questions where she knew he knew the answer. For example, she might ask, 'What should I do about the rent?' if she knew he would say 'pay it.' Of course if rent were a problem, she would not mention it. But a wife should let her husband feel like he is an active decision-maker." While these behavior tips are helpful, it is important not to continually put on an act. You must always be yourself.

* * *

"What is the best thing you can do for a person after a heart attack?" we asked a leading New York City psychiatrist.

"Reassure him," he said without hesitation. "Even if you turn out to be wrong." He continued, "I think this reassurance is vital. Some doctors hesitate because they are afraid they are giving too much encouragement. I think a person should be told they can resume all things in moderation, even if you are lying a bit. Most people prefer a good life even if it is shorter—and I am not saying it must necessarily be shorter—but I feel we should give the patient the greatest encouragement to be a vital, active person once again."

5. The Sexual Side

Is your sex life over? Absolutely not. After a heart attack, men do not become impotent, nor do they become sterile. They do not die suddenly during intercourse (except in very rare cases, and mainly those of extramarital sex).

"I asked my doctor what I should do about sex. All he said was 'Take it easy' " one patient complained. Doctors may be reluctant to discuss sex and patients may also be hesitant. "Truthfully, people just don't talk about it," a young cardiologist told us. "My patients just aren't asking, they seem to find it embarrassing."

Understanding sex is vital. It is a crucial part of resuming a normal life. The following cases are based on real people and real problems:

Case: Jerry, a fifty-four-year-old business executive, had an active sexual life with his young wife before his heart attack. After his attack, both were afraid to have sex. While neither said it directly, both feared that Jerry might suddenly die of a heart attack during intercourse.

Analysis: Sudden death is the most common fear and the most common myth about heart disease and sexuality. One cardiologist noted that intercourse was feared by his patients more than any other physical exertion. Sudden death during intercourse is very rare. One pathologist reported that out of 5,559 cases of sudden death, only thirty-four related to sexual activity. And twenty-seven of those deaths occurred during or after extramarital relations. Sudden death is extremely unusual when the heart patient engages in sex with a partner of many years.

"I've never seen a single patient in my practice who died during or immediately after intercourse," a noted cardiologist told us.

It should be noted that women can also suffer heart failure during sexual activity. Women are, however, less likely to be in such a situation. Although there are six women to every man over sixty-five, older women are not commonly taken as sexual partners by younger men.

Case: Walter was thirty-five when he had a sudden, massive heart attack on the tennis court. At the time, he and his wife were trying to have a child. After his recovery, Walter wondered if his wife would be able to conceive.

Analysis: Men do not become sterile after a heart attack. A man who has had a heart attack can sire a child. He will not be sterile unless he was sterile before.

If a woman has a heart attack while she is still ovulating (a rare occurrence), she will continue to ovulate and will continue to be able to have children.

It is worth noting that contraception should be practiced if children are not wanted. A heart attack offers no protection. For women with heart problems, however, the pill should be avoided. Other contraceptive methods should be discussed with the doctor.

Case: Mark, a seventy-year-old man, seldom had intercourse with his sixty-eight-year-old wife. After his heart attack, they stopped sexual relations altogether.

Analysis: Masters and Johnson have shown that people in their seventies and eighties can and do have sexual intercourse. However, desires vary. A general body response to any serious illness is loss of sexual desire. Many older men give up sex after a heart attack because they were about to give it up anyway. If this pattern is satisfying to them, that is fine.

Case: When George, age forty-eight, first had intercourse with his wife after his heart attack, he found he had many minor symptoms. He was aware of a rapid pulse, minor chest pain, and slight shortness of breath. He was worried and frightened by these symptoms.

Analysis: The first time intercourse is attempted after a heart attack, one might be acutely aware of unusual feelings. These symptoms are most common right after orgasm.

A landmark study by Doctors Hallerstein and Friedman showed that an awareness of excessively fast heartbeat was the most common complaint. Angina was next. For mild discomfort, many doctors recommend taking nitroglycerin before intercourse. This "before" pill usually relieves any discomfort.

Discomfort during intercourse the first time does not mean this discomfort will occur every time. Nor does it mean you are likely to provoke a heart attack with sex. With proper medication, sex can be safe and painless.

Case: John J., age thirty-four, had an active sex life before his heart attack. Although the doctor said he could resume intercourse, nonetheless John was nervous. He drank three double Scotches to ease his tension. Intercourse with his wife was not successful, and John feared he had become impotent.

Analysis: Alcohol does play an important role in successful sexual intercourse after a heart attack. Moderate amounts of alcohol will usually relax people. If there is an element of tension present that might hinder successful sexual relations, alcohol may be beneficial. For most men, however, an excess of alcohol will make it more difficult to achieve an erection and subsequently to complete the act. This may lead to prolonged foreplay and expending a great deal of effort attempting completion of intercourse. A brief, enjoyable experience may be turned into an exhausting marathon. Therefore alcohol intake must be limited.

Case: Henry suffered a minor heart attack shortly after he married for the second time. Since he was having sexual relations more frequently than he had in years, he feared this may have caused the attack. When Henry returned home, he and his wife were intimate and loving but were afraid to have intercourse.

Analysis: Intercourse does not cause heart attacks. Heart attacks build up over years and years. They are the result of a long-term, slowly developing disease process.

One of the myths of the June-December marriage is that the aged husband may die of heart failure, unable to keep up with the sexual demands of his young bride. This is not true. The percentage of heart attacks precipitated by sexual relations is, in fact, extremely low.

It is not a bad idea to be intimate without orgasm the first few times together. Dr. Joseph S. Alpert, formerly director of the Cardiac Unit at Peter Bent Brigham Hospital states, "It is a good idea to allow ample time for warm up (foreplay) remembering that the patient and his partner have been apart for a while." He also suggests "just being intimate without orgasm the first few times together—especially if either partner feels uneasy about resuming intercourse." After an adjustment period, however, intercourse can safely be resumed.

The amount of physical exertion required for sexual relations can almost always be tolerated without endangering the heart. Sexual relations with a spouse or usual partner are about as strenuous as briskly climbing two flights of stairs, or briskly walking a city block.

Case: John had diabetes and heart disease. As a result, he had become impotent. John wondered if he still could enjoy sexual foreplay, or would the frustration be too much strain for his heart.

Analysis: Sexual intercourse represents only a small segment of the total erotic experience. Sexual satisfaction can be obtained in many ways. Mutual holding, touching and caressing of the genitals, and oral genital sexuality can provide fulfilling outlets. These are safe practices and will not result in undue stress or tension.

Case: All the nurses knew Richard. He was the man who just had a heart attack but certainly didn't act it. He was always flirting, making seductive remarks, and he even tried to pinch a nurse.

Analysis: Sexual acting out is not unusual after a heart attack. It is a manifestation of aggressive sexual behavior. Psychologically, the person fears sexual impotence. This is compounded by forced dependency (on the young female nurses), loss of self-sufficiency, and loss of physical strength. These fears produce anxiety: The aggressive sexual behavior is an attempt to counteract this anxiety.

Psychiatric literature suggests that anxiety causes people to regress into an earlier, sexually immature level.

Case: John was married with three grown children. In the hospital, he met Nancy, an attractive divorced nurse. His wife was very upset by the situation. Nevertheless, John began dating Nancy, who was vibrant, sensual, and twenty years his junior. On attempting sexual intercourse, John felt intense pleasure but also intense pain. He thought he was going to die.

Analysis: Extramarital sex can be dangerous for the cardiac patient. Most deaths during intercourse occur during extramarital sexual encounters.

If a middle-aged man eats or drinks excessively and then attempts to perform sexually with a woman twenty years younger, he increases the risk of another heart attack or even death. "Death in the saddle," the name doctors give to this sex-related syndrome, occurs more frequently with a younger partner in an unfamiliar milieu.

Extramarital sex causes anxiety, guilt, and fear of detection. These factors may cause cardiac stress. Some authorities suggest that extramarital sex is more exciting, thus placing an extra burden on the heart. Whatever the reason, extramarital sex should be avoided by men who have had a heart attack.

Sexual Positions

A change in sexual position is sometimes recommended for heart attack victims so that the female can be the active partner.

The recommended intercourse positions are:

1. *Female superior (on top) intercourse position:*
   The patient lies on his back during intercourse with his partner sitting on top of him with her knees bent on either side. She is the active partner. This dependent supine position may be psychologically unacceptable to some men. If the man is the dominant, decision-making, controlling partner, using this position might upset him. If so, the customary male-on-top position should be used.

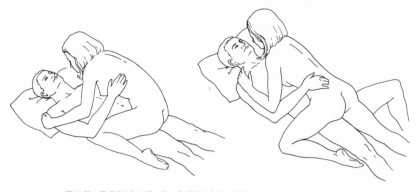

THE FEMALE SUPERIOR SEXUAL POSITION

After a heart attack, many doctors recommend the female superior intercourse position. In it, the woman has both knees touching the bed for traction. Thus, she is the active partner. If this is uncomfortable, doctors advise returning to what is most familiar.

2. *Lateral (side) intercourse position:*
   Couples often find it easiest to begin with the female superior position and then slide into this side position. From the sitting position, the woman slides one leg between the man's legs. In this way, she can have both knees touching the bed for traction. She is the active partner.
3. *Sitting intercourse position:*
   In this position, the couple sits in an armless chair facing each other. The wife sits on her husband's lap. The chair must be low enough so that both partners touch the floor with their feet. This position provides a maximum depth of penile penetration. Again, the wife is the active partner.

If these positions are difficult or awkward it is recommended to return to what is most comfortable. Many couples find this to be the male-on-top position. Because this position is the most common, a study was made to compare the cardiovascular stress in this male-on-top position with the male-on-bottom position. Ten healthy men, ages twenty-four to forty monitored themselves at home during intercourse. Each participant was requested to collect data during five periods of sexual activity: once for orientation, twice in the male-on-top position, and twice in the male-on-bottom position. The data showed that heart rate, blood pressure, and pressure-rate product (an indicator of myocardial oxygen uptake) were not significantly different in the two positions. The results of another study in middle-age males with arteriosclerotic heart disease by Doctors Hallerstein and Freidman showed similar results.

Impotence

You cannot become impotent from a heart attack. Fear, however, can cause impotence; a man can become psychologically impotent after a heart attack. Fear of failure, anxiety, or other emotional factors can make it difficult to have an erection.

No man can "will" an erection. It is an involuntary mechanism like breathing or heartbeat. Positive erotic feelings cause this sexual response.

The male sexual drive peaks at eighteen and declines thereafter. The middle-aged male requires more direct stimulation for penile erection. However, the ability to sustain an erection seems to be unaffected by aging. As a man gets older, ejaculatory release becomes less explosive, and less forceful penile contractions are perceived. With aging, some men require twelve to twenty-four hours before erection can be obtained again. A wife or partner should be aware of these factors.

Some heart pills can cause impotence. For example, a possible side effect of blood-pressure pills—Inderal, Lopressor, Ismelin, and Apresoline or Aldomet—may be impotence. Tranquilizers and anti-depressants may cause impotence or impaired ejaculation as a side effect. Men may complain of lack of interest in sex and difficulties in initiating and maintaining an erection. These are just possible side effects. Not every heart patient gets these drugs, and not every person who takes them becomes impotent.

Some forms of heart disease can also cause impotence. For example, if a man has diffuse atherosclerosis that is in the penis area, it may be difficult for him to have an erection. If this is the case, treatment is possible. There are now implants that can be surgically placed in the penis which make it possible to have an erection.

Masturbation

"I walked in and noticed a heart patient masturbating," a nurse reported. "Should I warn him against it? Is it dangerous?"

Masturbation is a normal sexual outlet. It is practiced by men from infancy to old age. It is also practiced by women but not as commonly.

Some doctors recommend that a return to sexual life begin with masturbation. They feel this is less demanding than intercourse. Recent studies at the University of Washington have reported that healthy young males, masturbating to the point of orgasm, experience a brief rise in cardiac rate to levels of 110 to 130 bpm. These rates are considerably lower than the tachycardia or 180 bpm, recorded in healthy young males during sexual intercourse.

Masturbation helps the patient gain sexual confidence. An erection provides visible proof that a man's masculinity remains intact.

During the convalescent stage when the patient is capable of walking a hall twice, masturbation should be considered an acceptable activity. A climate of acceptance from doctors, nurses, and family is important in relieving guilt or anxiety.

Gay sex

Gay men and gay women are not magically protected from heart attacks. They have heart attacks too. They can resume sexual activities after an attack.

Sexual Performance

Years ago, doctors warned against sex. They felt it involved too much physical and emotional strain and might precipitate another coronary. This has been completely disproved.

Today, sex is recommended. Dr. Eugene Scheimann states in

his book *Sex Can Save Your Heart . . . And Life,* "I strongly believe that a satisfying active sex life is the single most effective
protection against heart attacks that is available today . . . or
perhaps ever was." Sex releases tension and stress. It produces a
sense of well-being and creates a psychological closeness with one's
partner.

Sexual relations should resume gradually. "Initially couples
engage in mutual holding, touching and caressing without stimulation of the genitals," explains Rosalyn Jones Watts, Assistant
Professor at the University of Pennsylvania School of Nursing.
"After a few weeks, mutual stimulation of the breasts and genitals,
or, if acceptable, oral genital sexuality is added. Finally, sexual intercourse can be added to the sexual experience."

Most doctors say intercourse can be resumed three to eight
weeks after a heart attack.

Sex causes changes in the heart. Masters and Johnson report
that the blood pressure and heart rate increase. The heart rate increases from an average of 60 to 70 beats per minute to as many as
170 beats per minute with the average peak being 148.5 beats per
minute. The blood pressure rises from an average of 120/80 to as
high as 220/110 with the average being 170/100. Breathing may
rise to 60 breaths per minute. These changes last only one minute
and decline rapidly to normal within seconds after orgasm. Some
people have extra systoles or bursts of tachycardia.

For most people, these changes can easily be tolerated. Most
heart attack victims are middle-aged or older and sexual activity
in these age groups generally requires minimal physical exertion.

Oxygen consumption during orgasm in these people is less
than that required to walk briskly or to climb a flight of stairs.
Sexual activity of long-married couples, occurring on the average of
twice a week for relatively brief periods of time (ten to sixteen
minutes) requires no more energy than that required to participate
in an argument or drive a car.

Sexual intercourse with a spouse requires 5 to 6 Mets (meta-
bolic energy required). A man at rest requires 1 Met. The average
man can reach a level of 12 Mets, whereas the trained athlete can
attain a maximum capacity of 20 Mets. Most uncomplicated post-
myocardial heart patients can achieve a maximum of 9 Mets. The

energy expenditure before and after orgasm, that is during excitement, plateau, and resolution, is about 3.7 Mets. This knowledge of Met requirements for various sexual activities should give a person confidence in renewing sexual activity.

Possible Sexual Problems

Sex can, in certain people, cause heart strain. These are the warning signs:

- rapid heartbeat and rapid breathing persisting twenty to thirty minutes after intercourse
- palpitations continuing fifteen minutes after intercourse
- chest pain during or after intercourse
- sleeplessness following sexual activity
- an extremely "knocked out" feeling the day following intercourse

If any of these symptoms occur, check with your doctor before attempting sexual activity again. He may suggest one of the less active positions, less frequency, or limiting foreplay time, or he may give you pills. A long-acting form of nitroglycerin may be prescribed to be taken fifteen minutes before the sex act. This should be combined with a regular nitroglycerin tablet to be used two minutes before intercourse. Other drugs can also be used. These include propranolol, for extreme palpitations, and digitalis, for extreme shortness of breath. These usually ease completely any discomfort.

Sexual Warnings

Sex does put demands on the heart. Therefore, doctors warn that sexual relations should be avoided at these times:

- immediately after a large meal—wait at least two hours
- after drinking alcohol—a three-hour wait is advised
- just before or after strenuous activity
- if you are extremely anxious

- if you feel angry or resentful toward your partner
- if you are very tired
- if the environment is extremely cold or hot, especially when weather is hot and humid because of physiologic demands to maintain body temperature (in air-conditioned rooms is fine)

Just because a man has a heart attack, he doesn't suddenly become angelic. A man accustomed to extramarital sex may seek to prove he is still the same man he was. Indeed, a hitherto faithful husband may suddenly feel that he missed something. Recently Dr. Lenore Zohman, director of cardiopulmonary rehabilitation at New York's Montefiore Hospital stated "eight out of ten men who die during intercourse do so while engaging with partners other than their wives." It is important for men to be aware that extramarital sex can be dangerous for the man who has already suffered a heart attack.

Sexual Suggestions

Tension increases sexual problems. To enjoy sexual relations to their fullest, the following relaxation techniques may be helpful:

- play pleasant, restful, mood music
- meditate
- take a warm shower before sex
- drink a small glass of wine
- have sexual relations in the morning after a night's sleep (rest is more important *before* than after sexual relations)

What You Need to Know

A study by two leading cardiologists showed that two thirds of the heart attack patients surveyed had received no advice regarding sex; the rest had received nonspecific advice.

About one third had resumed normal sexual activity; two thirds had a marked and lasting decrease in the frequency of intercourse. Interviews suggested this change was based on misinformation and fear.

A man who has had a heart attack is *not* a sexual "has-been."

Myron Prinzmetal, one of the world's leading heart specialists, states, "There is no valid reason why the sex act should be avoided simply because the patient has had a coronary thrombosis. Once recovered, the person should be capable of precisely the same sexual frequency and style and intensity as before."

6. A Talk with Your Doctor

OVER HALF of all heart-attack victims go to their doctor within two weeks before their attack complaining of not feeling right. Yet the doctor finds no problem on the electrocardiogram and either gives another diagnosis, attributing symptoms to emotional factors, or issues a clean bill of health.

Diagnosing a heart attack *before* it occurs is immensely difficult, some say almost impossible. It is important to realize this and not blame the physician because a good doctor-patient relationship is extremely important.

A patient and doctor form a partnership during an illness. A warm and frank physician will bring feelings of reassurance and trust. A physician who does not establish rapport may cause distrust which can lead to further anxieties.

Many people fear their doctor; others worry they're wasting his time or—God forbid—they're boring him. Still others hold him in such high esteem, they can't communicate freely.

No relationship is perfect. "Sometimes I hate my husband's doctor and sometimes I love him," one wife confessed. While some people feel guilty about these emotions they are perfectly normal and understandable. Some people we spoke with had this to say about their doctor:

James Johnson, age forty-nine, after his first heart attack: "He could not have been nicer. I was very pleased with the doctor."

Jane Wilson, age fifty, after her husband's first heart attack: "I think every heart patient should have two cardiologists. Heart problems are so complex today, I think only one doctor is inadequate. Two heads are better than one. I just think two doctors will make fewer mistakes."

Jane Gotfried, age sixty, after her second heart attack: "I

just wouldn't have made it without him, not only medically, but emotionally too. When the tension seemed just too much, he seemed able to set things straight again."

Paul Dorsin, age thirty-two, after his second heart attack: "I wasn't pleased with the doctor. I wanted books. He just said 'go to the bookstore,' but he didn't have any specific suggestions. He didn't recommend counseling and I really wanted and needed it. He was vague, casual."

Jeffry Dags, age fifty-three, after his first heart attack: "The doctors prescribe, but the nurses really make you well. And you can quote me on that!"

How to Talk to Your Doctor

Good communication is the secret of a successful doctor-patient relationship. Unfortunately, many people are afraid to talk to their doctor. "They are so afraid, they actually whisper," Shelly Jacobson, a medical assistant in a Manhattan cardiologist's office said, "I'll tell you a typical story," she said. "Last week, an elderly woman came in.

" 'I've been having this heaviness in my chest for two weeks,' she whispered.

" 'Did you tell the doctor?' I asked.

" 'No,' she said.

" 'Why didn't you tell him?' I asked.

" 'I'm afraid,' she said.

"One woman told me worriedly, 'The doctor never tells me how the EKG looks.' I said, 'Do you ask him?' She said, 'No.' They are scared they might hear bad news so they just keep quiet and worry.

"Over 50 percent of the people we see here want to know about their condition but fail to understand it," Ms. Jacobson said.

How is it that two people—the doctor and the patient—with such an urgent need to communicate often fail? Emotions can block understanding. People are nervous about what ails them: They wonder if it's serious, if it's getting worse, if it will be painful or costly. They worry about missing work, and often they don't feel well.

Add to this the tempo of a busy doctor's office. If a doctor is interested in getting a person in and out of his office as quickly as possible, the person will feel this impatience.

Poor communication can impede the healing process. At times, it can be downright dangerous. Vague terms such as "use in moderation," "a few times a day," and "use your own discretion" frequently cause arguments. People will have varying interpretations. Wives may accuse husbands of "excessive nervousness," husbands may counter with "needless nagging."

Communication Hints

The following hints will help you communicate more effectively with your doctor:

1. Tell your doctor when you don't understand.
2. Write down his instructions.
3. Repeat them back to him, so you are sure you have them correctly.
4. Ask him about alternatives.
5. Practice what you want to say before the visit, write it down.
6. Breathe deeply before seeing the doctor to be as relaxed as possible.
7. Express your emotions honestly.

Unfortunately, some doctors, like some people, are basically insensitive. One wife told us, "We had a very bad experience with the residents. They were very pompous. I kept thinking, 'Don't they teach compassion in medical school anymore?' The whole hospital staff seemed to regard their work as just a nine-to-five job, and the doctors weren't any different."

The Office Visit

A heart attack often means the first time a person must regularly visit a doctor. Therefore, understanding the office visit is important. Basically, the office visit consists of a history, a physical examination, and a number of simple tests.

THE HISTORY. Your doctor will probably begin by talking with you and asking a series of questions about your present health and related factors. This is your "history." No amount of sophisticated technology, not even the computer, can replace this important form of human communication. A thorough history can provide 70 to 80 percent of the diagnosis; it can bring up and rule out various possible solutions and reveal which further tests need to be done. You can help your doctor take a good history by being as open and complete as possible.

The doctor will want to know what brought you to the office— what your chief complaint is—or if this is a routine visit. He or she will want to know the usual state of your health and what is different now. He or she will ask questions concerning all parts of your body from your eyes to your feet.

Because heart attacks tend to run in families, the doctor will also be interested in the health of your parents and other siblings.

In diagnosing and treating heart problems, your social history is also significant. So the doctor will ask you about the kind of work you do, your education, whether you smoke and how much, what kind of exercise you get, how is your diet and generally whether your life is stressful and how you handle it. Again, honesty is extremely important.

THE PHYSICAL EXAM. Next, the doctor will check your "vital signs"—your respiration, heart rate, and blood pressure. He will take your pulse (your heart rate is reflected in the expansions and contractions of an artery) and listen to your heart beat.

Auscultation. Auscultation is the act of listening to the sound within the body, usually with a stethoscope, to determine the condition of various organs beneath.

Taking the Pulse. Although the pulse is most commonly taken at one wrist, the doctor may compare the pulses in both wrists, the neck, the legs, and other locations as an indication of how good your peripheral circulation is, that is, circulation in areas of the body beyond the trunk.

Height and Weight. Height and weight are always measured since they can be an index of obesity. Overweight increases the risk of diabetes, high blood pressure, and therefore heart attacks.

Blood Pressure. It is very important that the doctor measure your blood pressure, the force of the flowing blood against the artery walls. This is taken with an instrument called a *sphygmomanometer* or blood pressure cuff.

Blood pressure is expressed by two numbers, for example

120/80 or 120 over 80. The higher number is the systolic pressure, the pressure each time the heart contracts. The lower number is the diastolic pressure, the pressure each time the heart relaxes.

You can't feel what your blood pressure is but a systolic of 140 or higher or a diastolic of 90 or higher can strain the heart and increase the risk of a heart attack. Fortunately, high blood pressure can be controlled.

SIMPLE HEART TESTS. As part of the office visit, the doctor will probably do some tests including:

A Blood Test. Doctors often take blood to test blood fat levels since high cholesterol and triglycerides increase the risk of clogged arteries. Blood tests also detect the presence of diabetes, another risk factor in developing heart problems.

EKG. The electrocardiogram (EKG or ECG) is given at almost every office visit for a heart patient. It can reveal irregular heart rhythms and also provides basic information on heart activity. It is completely painless.

Chest X Ray. A chest X ray is sometimes part of an office visit. X rays are useful in showing enlargement of the heart—very often one sign of a chronic heart problem and in detailing the circulation to the lungs.

What Specialist Is Needed?

Which doctor should you see after leaving the hospital? Experts suggest that you maintain contact with your primary physician, that is, your family physician (general practitioner) or internist.

The cardiologist is trained to concentrate on the cardiovascular system. Since you may have problems that have nothing to do with the heart, the cardiologist may not be the best equipped to be your primary physician. If, however, you have been cared for during your illness solely by the cardiologist, he could logically become your primary physician upon discharge if you wish.

Even if you are seeing your family doctor, it is advisable to visit your cardiologist at least twice a year, even if you are feeling marvelous. Your primary physician should be made aware of these consultations.

If you've had a heart attack, you've probably been examined by more medical specialists than you ever knew existed. To find out exactly what these various experts do, we spoke with them. Only their names have been changed so they could speak as openly and personally as possible.

A Cardiologist

Dr. David Rubanoff
Age: 36
Marital Status: married
Number of children: 2

A cardiologist is a physician who specializes in treating heart disease. His work begins when the family doctor finds something amiss, something that affects the heart, or when the patient is suddenly struck by a heart attack. After a heart attack, a cardiologist directs the medical care in the Coronary Care Unit and throughout the hospitalization. He also guides the patient in the post-heart-attack period.

Why did you become a cardiologist?

I took an elective in cardiology in my fourth year of medical school. The doctors I studied with made an art out of reading EKGs. I respected them greatly and I found the work fascinating.

Also I felt cardiac patients as a group were appreciative. Many heart diseases are treatable and the doctor's input can be significant.

How do you feel toward your patients?

I feel very sympathetic. Heart disease is a pervasive problem— it influences home and family life, work life, and financial matters. Patients become emotional. They may walk into the office looking fine, seemingly composed, but once they start talking, they often break down and cry. You must remain objective, but at the same time, you do not want to appear aloof. You must be compassionate and sympathetic; it is a difficult balance.

What advice do you give to wives?

Be patient. Your husband may be extremely up one day, extremely down the next. It takes time—several months—but things will even out and return to normal.

Remember, you are a human being too; speak up if you are being abused emotionally. If it persists, it's a red flag. You should not be embarrassed or ashamed to seek professional help. All wives find it an extremely difficult situation.

How often do you see patients who have had a heart attack after they leave the hospital?

I usually see patients ten days to two weeks after discharge from the hospital unless a problem develops sooner. Then I see them monthly for three months. If everything is fine, I then see them every two months, after that every four months and finally semiannually.

Even if they are feeling very well, it is important for all heart attack victims to be examined every six months.

What do you think is the most difficult thing in dealing with heart patients?

Heart patients are sick—sometimes very sick. They want and need help. Unfortunately, they must understand that medicine is not an exact science. Complications occur: Side effects occur. We are aware that they can occur but we do not know who will have them, who won't, and when they'll occur. It's hard if a patient takes a turn for the worse or if there are complications. Patients are suffering; it's tough to ask them to be understanding. I think this is the most difficult aspect of patient care.

How should a person feel toward his doctor?

A person should be very comfortable with his doctor. It is important that patients talk; it's funny but many don't. They should relate even the most minor symptoms—things they may feel are silly. The doctor can assess whether they are of note or not.

For example, a patient may be constipated . . . may have to strain, and be embarrassed to say so. However, this can be very significant. I had one patient who was transferred from the CCU, was very constipated from bed rest and analgesics. When he went to the toilet, he strained so much he ended up right back in the CCU.

It's very important that the doctor have time for the patient. He should answer all his questions so the patient understands everything as completely as possible.

Should a patient seek a second opinion?

That depends. Certainly a patient should feel free to see another specialist. Whether a second opinion is really necessary depends on the case. For a simple, uncomplicated heart attack, a person may not require a cardiologist. An internist or family doctor may handle the case and do an extremely competent job. If there is something unusual about the heart attack or if a complication develops, the doctor might call in a cardiologist.

Basically, if it makes a patient feel better at a difficult time, I'd say it's good to have an additional opinion.

What if a patient doesn't like his doctor?

If you don't like the doctor, and the reasons cannot be worked through, I think you should switch. For patients who are happy with their doctor, are doing well, and have known the doctor for a long time, I'd say "stay put." Don't be shoppers. Don't change horses in midstream.

A Psychiatrist

Dr. Jonathan Murphy
Age: 62
Marital Status: married
Number of children: 2   Number of grandchildren: 4

Seeing a psychiatrist is beneficial for everyone after a heart attack. It is not an admission of personal failure or weakness, but rather a needed treatment at a time of acute financial, social, and emotional stress.

In a recent British study, 143 men who had survived heart attacks were randomly divided into two groups: group one received intensive psychological counseling from the third day after the attack for six months; group two received the standard post-infarction advice.

As expected, those people with negative attitudes toward their illness and future did poorly regardless of the group they were in.

People assessed as being neurotic and introverted had a significantly poorer outcome in the standard group compared with similar people in the psychologically oriented group. And people in the psychological counseling group returned to work in greater numbers and sooner than did those in the control group and showed greater physical and emotional stability and greater social independence.

Who should see a psychiatrist after a heart attack?

Everyone can benefit from speaking to a psychiatrist after a heart attack. There cannot be a heart attack without emotional complications. Someone must deal with these emotional difficulties, but it does not have to be a psychiatrist, per se. An internist, cardiologist, social worker, or psychologist can act as the therapist.

When should the therapy begin?

This depends on the emotional reaction to the heart attack. People who become obviously anxious and depressed should see a therapist quickly. For those not so obvious problems, some sessions would be beneficial after discharge when the person is beginning to resume normal life.

How does a person who has had a heart attack know if he needs therapy?

If the person finds himself fearful of the future, preoccupied with anxious thoughts and fantasies, such as fear of death, or if the person has frequent nightmares, feels tense, depressed, or believes the quality of his life is forever impaired—then he should think in terms of seeing a psychiatrist.

Should a wife go too?

This is not normally necessary. However, wives must be educated about their husband's disease. One of the most important things for a wife to avoid is making her husband a "cardiac cripple." If the wife is fearful, the husband will pick up on it. Fear can be more destructive than heart disease. Wives must be taught that men should resume normal living as soon as possible.

How can a wife open communications with a silent husband?

This is difficult. Some people simply will not talk. They do not like to share confidences; they feel it is evidence of weakness. They are the "I'll do it myself" or "I don't need any help" types. The wife may feel shut out and there may be little she can do to open communication.

However, more commonly, people are ashamed to admit fears and feelings. For this type of person you might try saying, "I know you're thinking this," or "I know you're afraid of . . ." or "I know you're worried about . . . ." This will give them a chance to open up and verbalize their feelings.

Will talking make things worse and cause arguments?

I think that's just a rationalization. When there are problems rumbling around, it is always helpful to bring them to the surface.

If you don't talk about a problem, it still exists. The subject may not be discussed but it is nonetheless upsetting. In fact, it's more destructive in the preconscious state than when it's brought to the surface. Talking lessens the impact of worries.

Can antidepressant drugs be taken by heart attack victims?

Yes, cautiously, under a doctor's supervision. Some types are more cardiotoxic than others.

Can lithium be given safely?
Yes.

Is shock therapy safe after a heart attack?
With precautions, it can be done safely.

What about tranquilizers?

Tranquilizers are given routinely to people immediately after a heart attack. Almost every patient is given Valium or a similar sedative agent.

What can be done for overt hostility and anger?

There are medications. More importantly, it is essential to find out why the person is angry and deal with the causes. If the husband is angry because he feels his wife created conditions which pressured him and therefore led to the attack, both partners must understand these feelings. Some people are just angry; they are angry with God. Again, we must expose this anger to reason and logic. Most people are angry they got sick. We must explain that as human beings these are the risks and we can cut down the risks somewhat, but we cannot become divine.

What do you recommend for excessive nervousness?

This is not easily controlled and seeing a psychiatrist would be helpful. There are many reasons for nervousness. For example, some people feel they were bad children. They are perpetually anxious, worried that the axe will fall. Usually this is an individual problem best handled on a personal basis.

What is the best way of dealing with the children?

I think it's best if the person who had the heart attack talks with the children and reassures them. You must assume the children have some worries. The person who had the heart attack is the best one to tell them, "We're going to do everything we always did." It's also appropriate for the doctor to make an effort to speak with the children.

Should a wife try to get her husband to see a psychiatrist even if he is resistant?

Yes. She should gently suggest it from time to time.

What "difficult" period can be expected? When does this become abnormal?

It's almost universal that the first psychological response after a heart attack is anxiety with fear of dying. When that subsides within a few days, there is always a depressive reaction which has to do with "I'm not going to be the same guy I was." That lasts about a week or two. If it lasts longer or if anxiety continues longer than a few days, it is no longer a normal reaction and some steps should be taken. Depression and anxiety snowball, so prompt treatment is important.

What is the most important thing in dealing with a person after a heart attack?

I think the key word is support. The family, friends, and professionals must give a great deal of reassurance, I feel, even if the future is not totally clear.

For the wife I think the most important thing is conquering irrational fear. Excessive caution can be psychologically dangerous. It can turn men into cardiac cripples.

A Physiatrist

Dr. Saul Mortimer
Age: 54
Marital status: single
Children: none

A physiatrist is a physician who specializes in rehabilitation medicine. He cares for people after strokes, arthritis, and other debilitating diseases. A physiatrist literally helps people get back on their feet. Heart attack patients are rarely this disabled, but sometimes, if they feel very weakened, the services of a physiatrist during a hospital stay is helpful.

How do the patients you see feel?

They are always frightened, fearful it will happen again. They say, "Look, this happened to me once and it could happen again any time." So they are afraid to walk, afraid to talk, sometimes even to eat.

Some patients are very hostile—the "so what are *you* going to do?" attitude. Others go to the opposite helpless extreme—the "do you think I'll ever get better?" attitude.

What is your role?

We try to put them slowly back on a daily routine. We show them they can walk. If they were active before, we try to eventually go to where they were before.

Does the patient or his family call you?

No. A cardiologist or another physician asks the physiatrist to see the patient.

Generally, "rehab doctors" work only in hospitals and nursing homes. There is no private office; therapy takes place during the hospitalization.

How does the rehabilitation program begin?

The cardiologist usually calls me in a day or two after the person leaves the CCU. First I'll take a detailed history. I find out what the patient's life was like before the attack. How active were they?

Then I'll begin working at the edge of their bed. I'll tell them to dangle their legs at the side. Then I'll show them how to stretch their legs and stretch their arms. I emphasize if they feel angina or dizziness or nauseated or short of breath to stop immediately. Usually they start deep breathing, hyperventilating because they are afraid. We show them how to breathe normally.

I remind them to always keep their eyes open so they don't faint. I exercise them on the bed for a day or two. Then I have them walk to their chair, then down the hall, and then around the nursing station several times a day. Gradually I have them do more and more.

How often do you see the patients?

At first twice or three times a week, then about once a week. It depends on the person and the heart attack.

What do the heart attack patients tell you?

They'll say "Why me?" That's the first thing they always say. I tell them illness doesn't consider who, what, when and where. I tell them it is sometimes a timely warning to look at their lives—still enjoy, but live sensibly.

What do wives say?

The wives are often speaking for their husbands. I like to interview the men alone.

Wives will say—"Now tell him if he doesn't do it he'll get

worse." Of course, this is not always the best approach. Sometimes you have to be very tough with people, but I try all approaches, depending on the person.

What is the biggest difficulty in dealing with these people?

Many heart attack patients don't want to accept something is wrong. The men say, "I have to support my family. I have to continue working." It's hard to make them slow down.

What is your greatest frustration in dealing with heart patients?

When I know someone can do something and he just doesn't want to. I try every method I can—I am coarse; I am tough; I try being nice. I am understanding and try to show him he can do it, but if he doesn't want to help himself, it's impossible to make him.

Are women more cooperative than men?

No. The men in their forties, fifties and early sixties seem to do the best. Once people reach the middle sixties, it's more difficult.

What about the younger person?

They have one of two reactions. Either they say this can't happen again, or they quit everything and say I can't do anything because it *will* happen again.

What about the geriatric patient?

The older person generally just sits around and mopes. Many older people would rather be invalids.

Is there any difference in attitude between rich and poor patients?

Rich or poor doesn't make any difference at all. I had one well-to-do woman who said, "Get the ——— out of my life." She wouldn't move because I wouldn't feel sorry for her. On the other hand, some wealthy people have terrific drive. You just can't generalize.

What advice do you give to families?

Be active. Almost any exercise is good. Start walking. Remember we have two legs; use them.

A Cardiac Surgeon

Stephen Senduranu
Age: 40
Marital status: married
Number of children: none

A cardiac surgeon performs surgical operations on parts of the heart. The most commonly done operation for heart-attack victims is coronary bypass surgery. It is occasionally performed on people who have had recent heart attacks. Usually two to three months are allowed to elapse between a heart attack and cardiac surgery.

What is the training of a cardiac surgeon?

First they must be fully trained general surgeons. This means four years of medical school, one year internship, and four years of residency in surgery. For cardiac surgery, an additional two years of thoracic and cardiovascular training is required. A cardiac surgeon must have double certification. He must be certified by the American Board of Surgery. After passing this examination, he must then be examined by the American Board of Thoracic Surgery.

Who should see a cardiac surgeon?

A person should be referred to a cardiac surgeon by a cardiologist or internist.

Today, some patients hear about bypass surgery and they call the surgeon directly. This is not the best route. The surgeon will usually send him to be evaluated by a cardiologist first, in any case.

Who should have bypass surgery?

The indications for bypass surgery are complicated, but in general, it is recommended if the person is unresponsive to medical treatment, and/or has significant multivessel or main left coronary artery disease.

If the person has a lot of anginal pain, we can often give him enough medicine to guarantee a pain-free existence. But he may have to be so medicated that it is difficult to work or drive, so quality of life is another consideration.

What is the cost of bypass surgery?

About $12,000 to $15,000.

How long does the operation take?

It depends of course, but generally, the operation will take three to four hours.

How long does the patient stay in the hospital?

An average of about ten days. Generally, two months after surgery they can return to work.

Should all people who have a heart attack consider coronary artery surgery?

Not at all. Many people who have a heart attack never develop angina. They would neither need nor benefit from surgery.

Do all patients who need surgery require cardiac catheterization?

Absolutely. This is a guide for the surgeon and helps identify with precision abnormal areas in the heart chambers and arteries.

Does catheterization have risks?

Yes, there are risks and they should be clearly understood.

Psychologically, how do people cope with bypass surgery?

Before surgery, there is always anxiety. People wonder, why is he recommending surgery? Is he right? Do I really need it? Wives worry, "Am I doing the right thing in taking my husband to this surgeon?" But after surgery, the person usually improves markedly and these worries are forgotten.

Do most people see it as a quick cure?

Most people are not eager for surgery, but a few are. I saw a forty-three-year-old shipbuilding engineer with angina. All he wanted to do was get back to skiing. He didn't believe in medicines. He viewed surgery as a panacea. And for him it has been! He's off all medicines—except aspirin—jogging two-and-one-half miles a day, and skiing spring and winter.

If angina was a problem before, will it be cured by surgery?

Studies show in over 90 percent of patients, angina is relieved by surgery. Some people still have angina but it is less severe. One construction worker I operated on insisted he developed arthritis after the operation. I've told him it's angina but he says it's nothing like he had before.

Will shortness of breath be cured?

Shortness of breath is usually not helped by this operation.

Can atherosclerotic narrowings be removed surgically?

No, such narrowings cannot be removed, but they can be bypassed to enable the blood to get to the heart muscle.

Another method of dealing with this problem is a new procedure, still considered developmental, called transluminal coronary angioplasty. In this procedure, a balloon-type catheter is inserted into the diseased coronary artery where it presses the atherosclerotic plaque back against the coronary artery wall, thereby increasing the blood flow. More will be learned about this procedure in the coming years.

A CCU Nurse

Marilyn Jones
Age: 46
Marital status: married
Number of children: 2 teenagers

All the people we interviewed expressed such praise for the nurses in the Cardiac Care Units, we felt their experiences and expertise should be included in this chapter.

Do the CCU nurses have special training?

Yes. All the nurses in the unit are R.N.'s. In addition, they have all completed a four-week, full-time, critical-care course given at the hospital. All nurses, even experienced nurses who have worked in other CCU's, must go through the course.

How large is your unit?

Our hospital has an eight-bed unit; each patient has his own room. There are thirteen nurses working around the clock. One doctor sleeps in the unit.

What is the nurse/patient ratio?

In the CCU, there is one nurse for every three to four patients. On a regular hospital floor, there is one nurse to about twelve patients. If a CCU patient is critically ill, there might be one nurse for one patient.

Are private-duty nurses necessary?

Private-duty nurses are not allowed in the Coronary Care Unit. On the regular floor, these nurses are permitted. In most cases, they are not needed.

How long do the patients stay in the CCU?

If they have had a heart attack and have no complications, they'll stay five days. If they are there for observation, they'll stay three days.

How many of the patients in the CCU have had heart attacks before?

About one in three. The rest are there as a preventative or observation measure, perhaps because they've had irregular rhythms or chest pains.

Who is your typical patient?

He's male, married, a white-collar worker, in his mid-sixties.

We do get some women. Interestingly, they are generally younger than the men. They're usually in their fifties.

What is the biggest physical problem for the patients?

Having a bowel movement. They seem preoccupied with it. We tell them they won't have a bowel movement for two to three days because of changes in their diet and surroundings. We allow them to go use a commode rather than a bedpan because we feel it is more comfortable. Interestingly, it is less energy-taxing than using a bedpan.

What is the biggest emotional problem?

While the patients are lying in bed, they seem to reflect on their lives. They become very, very passive and dependent. They don't verbalize their feelings; it is too soon. I think the nurses on the regular floors hear more.

In fact, they don't even ask if it was a heart attack. For the first two days, it is still an unknown factor. Generally the families ask but the patient doesn't.

Is any counseling offered in the unit?

I never had a patient who requested counseling. If the patient has complete denial, if he's threatening to sign out or if he seems confused, we might suggest it to the physician.

How does the patient look?

They look much better than most people expect. We see families walking into the room hesitantly as if they don't know what to expect. Generally, the patients don't look sick. The crisis is usually passed. They may read a newspaper, watch TV or sit in a chair. They nap on and off. We don't want them to sleep all the time. If we see they are sleeping too much, we will cut back on the sedation.

How does the monitoring work?

There are painless leads on the chest. The EKG machine is in the room; it is connected to a central hookup at the nurses' station. It looks like a TV screen. A nurse is observing it at all times. If there is any irregularity, an alarm system is activated. A light flashes, a buzzer sounds, and a cardiogram begins to write.

How do patients feel if another patient has a cardiac arrest?

Of course they know; they see a flurry of activity. But each patient is in a separate room. As long as they are separated by the walls, they feel protected. They ask, of course, yet it doesn't seem to affect them personally.

What is the atmosphere in the CCU?

We try to make it very comfortable and informal. All the nurses are called by their first names, and we assign the same nurse to the same patient throughout the day.

Do CCU nurses make more money?

No. All nurses in the hospital receive the same salary.

Do nurses like working in the CCU?

Yes, it is a very prestigious job in nursing. There is a tremendous amount of job satisfaction. You get a great deal of recognition as part of the health team. These nurses can make an immense—indeed lifesaving—difference and they know it.

Of course, when the nurses first come into the unit, they are scared. But with supervision and direction they grow into the responsibilities. The nurses like it and they stay for years. There are very few staff changes.

Is there anything the patients should know when they leave the CCU?

The patients are so dependent that leaving the unit can sometimes be difficult for them. We assure them they are ready to be transferred, they will be okay without the monitor. They are a little anxious, feeling that they are suddenly thrown on their own. For the first few days, it can be difficult.

What is most rewarding about your job?

There is a very close rapport with the patient. You meet his family. You learn his emotional as well as physical problems, and you can really help with both at a time of crisis.

What is most difficult about your job?

Coping with your own anxiety. When the patient is in a very critical condition, you're waiting and watching to see if something will happen. You must have keen observation. Once something happens, it is not as difficult. Then you do what has to be done. But there is anxiety beforehand, wondering what will happen.

Have the patients or treatments changed throughout the years?

Yes, tremendously. Years ago, we had them lying like zombies for weeks. Today, we let them know they're alive and not incapacitated. They can feed themselves. Twenty-four hours after the attack, they are sitting up in a chair. They can watch TV, read a newspaper.

Today, it's okay to verbalize emotions, but years ago, that component wasn't recognized. Today, if you want to cry, it's okay. Years ago, everything was hidden.

During an illness a doctor and a patient form a partnership. It is the combined efforts of the patient and the doctor that results in a happy outcome. A famous physician once said, "The cure of an illness is 50 percent in the hands of the Lord, 49 percent in the trust the patient has in his physician and perhaps 1 percent in his physician's skillful care."

It is essential that a person be happy with his physician. If he is not, he should switch.

Too often, patients stay in unhappy relationships with their doctor. Some people feel their medical histories are so complex, a new doctor would be unable to "come in the middle." This just is not so. By looking at previous hospital and office records, a new physician can know a complete medical history. There is no situation so complicated that a person should feel a new doctor cannot be called in.

Everyone likes recognition. Although a doctor gets a fee, he still likes to know that the care he's rendering is being appreciated. No formal thank you, no reverential worship, but a general sense of appreciation is important. And, in turn, your doctor can help set the stage, emotionally and physically, for a new, healthier lifestyle.

7. Sources of Help

No family needs to be reminded of the stresses after a heart attack. But families do need to be reminded of how and where they can find help. The following sources can help with financial, social, and emotional problems in the post-heart-attack period.

Get Help Fast

We have already said it. But it bears repeating. AFTER A HEART ATTACK, GET HELP QUICKLY. A delay of a few moments can mean the difference between life and death.

Don't hesitate to call the doctor or worry about disturbing him. Don't wait until he calls back. Get yourself to the emergency room of a hospital fast.

Alarming Symptoms that Require Immediate Response

- severe chest pain lasting more than ten minutes
- sudden rapid pulse rate
- irregular pulse, particularly very slow pulse
- sudden acute nausea and vomiting

Believe it or not, some people are too embarrassed to ask for help. Recently, a CPA called his cardiologist saying he had severe pain in his shoulder that just would not go away. The doctor asked if he had taken nitroglycerin. No he said, because he was embarrassed to appear sick in front of a client. When the doctor urged him to get to the hospital, he asked, "What can I tell my client?"

Many people do not realize an emergency is occurring. An emergency ambulance dispatcher gave us the following account: "A young man was mowing his lawn on a hot summer day. He came into the house complaining of crushing chest pain. His wife gave him an aspirin and told him to take a nap. He couldn't sleep because of the pain and started pacing the floor rubbing his left arm. His wife gave him some brandy and said she would lie down with him. When she went to awaken him, she couldn't. Immediately she called the ambulance. Unfortunately, it was too late. The man had already died of a heart attack.

"People must be aware of cardiac symptoms and cardiac emergencies," this dispatcher told us. "Our biggest problem is people wait too long."

Ten years ago, even if you reached the hospital in the first hour after your heart attack, you still had a 30 percent chance of dying. Today, if you get to a hospital quickly, the mortality rate is only 15 percent.

In some cases, getting to the hospital is not enough. You must insist on being treated promptly. "We waited five hours in the emergency room before we were finally taken," one woman told us. "That night, the hospital called and said my father had died of a heart attack. We are bitter. I still think, if they had helped him sooner, maybe things would have worked out differently."

Help in the Hospital

Besides medical care, hospitals also offer help for the family. The following professionals can provide meaningful guidance.

THE HOSPITAL SOCIAL WORKER. A social worker is trained to help patients verbalize their anxiety during this difficult period. They also provide concrete services. For example, they can provide referral to the office of vocational rehabilitation, they can assess the home situation and arrange for homemakers if needed. They can assist in solving transportation problems. A social worker can be contacted directly by a patient or his family. Sometimes the nurse on the floor or physician will bring the person to the attention of the social service department.

THE HOSPITAL CHAPLAIN. The hospital chaplain can provide

comfort for the victim, his spouse, and family during a difficult hospitalization. The chaplain's role is to provide spiritual guidance, but not in a strictly religious sense. He probably will not read prayers or scripture (although if you wish, he certainly would) but rather he will help you struggle with questions about life and life's meaning at a time of crisis.

THE OCCUPATIONAL THERAPIST. The occupational therapist shows the person less stressful ways of performing the activities of daily living. They provide ideas for making kitchen chores easier, for example, putting commonly used things at waist level to save bending, arranging all cooking ingredients first to save steps, using a stool to lessen standing and using a wheeled cart for transporting food to and from the table.

A visit by the occupational therapist must be requested by a physician. Either the psychiatrist, cardiologist, or internist usually makes the referral. The occupational therapist usually sees the person twice a week, sometimes three times depending on individual needs. Occupational therapists do *not* do job counseling.

Services Outside the Hospital

Many services are available in the months and even years after your heart attack. Some are available only through direct referral by your physician.

How much help you need depends on your recovery. The size of a heart attack, rate of healing, and general strength vary from person to person. Consequently, the time it takes to recuperate after a heart attack will vary also. A previously healthy individual who suffers a small heart attack might return to full activity within four to six weeks. On the other hand, a person having a larger heart attack or one experiencing other health problems may require a convalescent period of three to six months. After two to three months, most people will be able to return to their previous work and recreation levels.

A few of the services offered to families are listed below. While these are found in the New York City area, most areas offer similar services. These can be found in your telephone directory under the given title.

Financial Assistance

Department of Social Services, City of New York
250 Church Street
New York, N.Y.   10013

(*Note:* Similar services are available in all cities, look in your directory under Department of Social Services)

Federal Disability Insurance
Department of Health, Education and Welfare
Washington, D.C.

Provides information concerning eligibility for Medicare disability benefits. Contact your local social security office. The address and telephone number are listed in the directory under Social Security and Medicare.

State Workmen's Compensation
2 World Trade Center
New York, N.Y.   10047
Tel: (212) 488-4141

Most laws provide that any heart attack suffered during or within a reasonable period after an unusual physical exertion or mental strain at work will be compensated.

These situations are presumed to have precipitated the heart attack. This board also provides information about benefits to replace, in part, wages lost by workers disabled *off-the-job.*

Housing Help

NYCHA (New York City Housing Authority)
250 Broadway
New York, N.Y.   10007
Tel: (212) 233-2525

Provides information on public housing, particularly if you must relocate to a ground floor or elevator building because of continuing heart problems.

Home-Care Services

Information Bureau
Community Council of Greater New York
225 Park Avenue South
New York, N.Y.   10003
Tel: (212) 777-5000

Provides information on home health attendants and gives telephone reassurance.

VNS
Visiting Nurse Service
107 East 70th Street
New York, N.Y.
Tel: (212) 535-9520

Referral is by head nurse on patient's floor, or by physician or social worker *before* hospital discharge. Provides part-time nursing care, physical therapy, and home health aide service. The fee is adjusted according to the family income.

Social Security Administration Office
39 Broadway
New York, N.Y.
For Manhattan Tel: (212) 432-3232

Each borough in New York has its own offices. Each city in the U.S. has an office. It offers information concerning home care services provided by Medicare.

New York City Department of Social Services
Long-Term Home Health Care Program
330 West 34th St.
New York, N.Y.
Tel: (212) 971-2675

Provides information concerning home care services provided by the New York City Department of Social Services (Medicaid). Every large city has a Medicaid (public assistance) office.

Nursing Sisters, Sister's Home Visiting Services, Inc.
310 Prospect Park West
Brooklyn, N.Y.   11215
Tel: (212) 965-7345

Provides part-time skilled nursing care in the home as well as physical therapy. Has a sliding scale of fees and accepts some third-party reimbursement.

Physical Rehabilitation

Your local YMCA or YMHA

Most local Y's now provide cardiac rehabilitation under the supervision of a doctor or nurse. These individually tailored programs are based on stress tests. Participants must be at least three months post heart attack.

Employment Assistance

Most large companies and organizations as well as police and fire departments have a program where workers are evaluated and assisted as necessary.

Office of Vocational Rehabilitation
New York State Education Department
225 Park Avenue South
New York, N.Y.   10003
Tel: (212) 777-7010

Provides vocational rehabilitation services, including vocational counseling, training, and placement.

B'nai B'rith Career Counseling Services
823 UN Plaza
New York, N.Y.
Tel: (212) 490-0677

For members and relatives of members, they offer assistance in career choice as well as second-career and pre-retirement counseling. There is a fee.

Federation Employment and Guidance Service
215 Park Ave. South
New York, N.Y.   10010
Tel: (212) 777-4900

Provides job placement, vocational guidance, vocational re-habilitation services, skills, training remediation, and job-related education. Also includes testing when necessary. Fee based on a sliding scale.

Self-Help Groups
Self-help groups are very active and immensely helpful for heart-attack victims and their families. As one 54-year-old woman who had bypass surgery told us, "These people know what the experience really is like. No doctor can imagine it; the support you get is indescribable."

To contact the heart club in your area, ask your physician, the hospital social worker, or your local heart association chapter.

Educational and Recreational Opportunities
Board of Education of the City of New York
Office of Continuing Education
110 Livingston Street
Brooklyn, N.Y.   11201
Tel: (212) 596-5030

Provides fundamental adult education and high school equivalency courses.

Your Local Library

Libraries provide excellent information on educational and recreational programs offered by public and voluntary agencies. They can also suggest pertinent reading material after a heart attack.

General Guidance
United Neighborhood Houses of New York
101 E. 15th Street
New York, N.Y.   10010
Tel: (212) 677-0300

Provides information about and referral to other community agencies in the greater New York area.

U.S. Government Printing Office
26 Federal Plaza
New York, N.Y.   10007
Tel: (212) 264-3826

Provides free and inexpensive brochures on heart disease, diet, and government assistance programs.

Literature and General Information

American Heart Association
Dallas, Texas (National Office)

Chapters within each state. For example:

New York Heart Association
205 East 42nd Street
New York, N.Y.
Tel: (212) 661-5335

Lenox Hill Hospital
Health Education Center
110 East 77th Street
New York, N.Y.   10017
Tel: (212) 794-4515

They do not send out general information but can provide information on specific health problems.

Center for Medical Consumer and Health Care Information, Inc.
237 Thompson Street
New York, N.Y.
Tel: (212) 674-7100

Provides information via tapes over the telephone. They will also send general information if you send them a self-addressed stamped envelope.

NYC Department of Health: Heart Beat
Tel: (212) 431-4540
Spanish Heart Beat: Tel: (212) 431-4558

Each week they have a different tape, usually related to heart problems and diet. Tapes in Spanish are also offered.

CPR Can Help

Doctors recommend that at least one family member (and preferably two) learn cardiopulmonary resuscitation (CPR).

It is a relatively simple procedure. Classes are given under the auspices of all local Heart Association chapters, local branches of the American Red Cross and many hospitals. CPR should be performed only by those who have completed the course.

CPR is used before an ambulance or rescue squad arrives. It involves artificial respiration and external cardiac compression. It is best performed by two people.

One person should administer artificial respiration, the other should apply external cardiac compression. Coordination of the two efforts is required. If one person must do two jobs, it is difficult but not impossible.

Here are the basic emergency resuscitation steps. (CPR cannot be learned from a book. These steps are provided as reminders for those who have already taken the course.)

1. Attempt to arouse the victim; if that is not possible, tilt head back, opening the airway. Look, listen, and feel for breathing. If the person is breathing, do nothing but summon help to get the victim medical attention as fast as possible. Call the police or fire department if transportation is a problem. Keep the airway open.
2. If there is no breathing, pinch the nostrils and form a tight seal over the victim's mouth. Give four quick breaths of air into the person. Do not pause between breaths.
3. If you cannot breathe into the victim, reposition the head and try again. Should you fail again, execute the obstructed airway maneuver. (Review this with your CPR instructor.)
4. After four quick successful breaths, feel the carotid pulses. If they are present but the victim doesn't breathe on his own, continue rescue breathing, with the airway opened, once each five seconds.

5. If pulses are absent, begin chest compression by placing the palm of one hand on lower portion of the breast bone, the other palm over it. Keep your elbows stiff and compress the chest down one-and-one-half to two inches. If you are alone, press down each time you say a number in the phrase, "One and two and three and four and five and" for three cycles then go back to the head, tilt it, and breathe twice. If two rescuers are present, press one time for each second saying, "One one-thousand, two one-thousand, three one-thousand . . ." The other rescuer breathes each time you get to, "five one-thousand."

6. Continue to alternate between compression and breathing. Every four cycles, recheck the carotid pulses to determine if independent circulation has returned. Failing to find pulses, continue CPR.

7. After each breath remember to take your mouth away to permit air to be exhaled.

8. Continue this method until it is taken over by another rescuer, ambulance or emergency medical personnel, or physician.

While researching this chapter, we were disappointed to learn about the limited services available to people after a heart attack. "After leaving the hospital, that was it," one man said. "You were completely on your own. And really that was the toughest time—the time you really needed help."

A wife of a heart victim said, "I would have loved a group session with other wives but no one suggested it."

A heart attack is a time of crisis. Everyone needs help. Unfortunately, you must actively seek assistance. But there are services—and many are free—which can give the family understanding and concrete suggestions at this difficult time.

PART TWO

Medical Facts

8. A Look at Your Heart

"I GUESS I'm so worried because it's the heart. I mean the *heart*. You can live without one eye, one ear, but the *heart*. That's it," one concerned wife told us.

"It's all so sudden and so irrational," said the daughter of a man who suffered his first heart attack during a hospitalization for a prostate operation. "When a person is in the hospital with all that equipment, you just don't think they should suddenly have a heart attack. At least with cancer, you know it's there. It's progressive and it's terminal. But in heart attacks, some survive, some don't; no one seems to know which it will be until it happens."

Anatomy lessons are sometimes boring. But when something has happened to your own heart or that of a loved one, you are suddenly very interested. Nothing about the heart is dull anymore because it affects you—every day of your life.

To better understand what may go wrong and why, you must first understand the basic workings of the human heart.

A Miraculous Machine

No man-made machine—no matter how complex—can compare with the miraculous workings of the human heart.

Your heart begins beating before your birth and continues unceasingly for seventy or eighty years. If for any reason it should stop for more than four minutes, you would die.

Did you realize that the heart:

· pumps 10 pints of blood each minute
· beats 60 or 70 times a minute

- pumps up to 6½ gallons per minute in heavy exercise
- pumps about 3,000 gallons of blood every day

Your heart does this monumental amount of work yet it is only the size of your fist and weighs less than one pound!

The heart pumps blood. The blood carries oxygen and nutrients to all the organs of your body. At the same time, the blood removes excess by-products, water, and carbon dioxide.

The blood reaches the body organs through a vast network of blood vessels. Should all these blood vessels be joined end to end, they would reach almost 2½ times around the earth—some 60,000 miles. *And* the heart pumps blood through this vast network and back to the heart in approximately ten seconds!

Even more amazing, the blood does not flow at a constant rate through all your organs but adapts, depending on the conditions in each organ at a given moment. For instance, when you jog, the blood flow to your leg muscles quickly increases through the dilation of the blood vessels in your legs. At the same time, the flow to

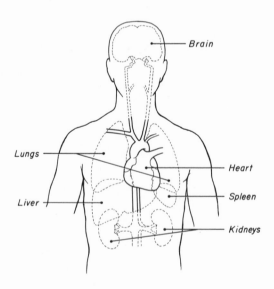

THE HEART WITH OTHER BODY ORGANS

About the size of your fist and weighing less than a pound, the heart is the organ on which all others depend.

less active areas decreases. Likewise, when you eat a large meal, there is a proportionately greater flow to the intestines; when you study, the brain receives more blood.

Nature Protects the Heart

The heart does not just hang freely on the chest. Around it is a loose, fluid-filled, protective sack of tissue called the *pericardium*. This sack is loose enough to permit the heart to beat easily.

Directly along the surface of the heart is a thin, shiny membrane called the *epicardium.*

The largest part of the heart is a thick mass of muscle called *myocardium*. This is the actual working part of the heart. The myocardium is thickest in the left ventricle (this pumps blood to the whole body); it is thinnest in the atria (this just stores the blood).

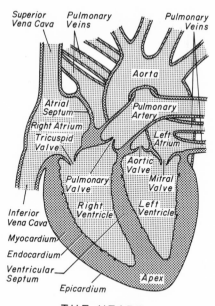

THE HEART

The heart is a miraculous muscle, beating about seventy times a minute, day and night, for a lifetime.

The inside of the heart is also protected by a lining. This thin, smooth membrane called the *endocardium* also covers the heart valves.

Parts of the Heart

Your heart has four chambers. Each of the top chambers is called an *atrium*. This comes from the Latin meaning "porch." These small thin-walled chambers act like entry rooms to the great chambers below. They are the collecting chambers.

The *ventricles* are thick-walled chambers that do the real work of pumping blood. These chambers form the great mass of the heart.

Down the middle of the heart is a thick wall. Much like the nose, the *septum* divides the heart into right and left parts. The important thing to remember about this wall or septum is that it is absolutely watertight, or more accurately, bloodtight. No blood can pass through this septum from one side of the heart to the other.

Each side of the heart has a different function. The right side of the heart collects blood from the body and pumps it to the lungs. The left side of the heart collects blood from the lungs and pumps it to the body.

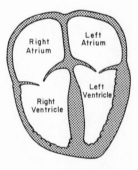

THE HEART'S CHAMBERS

The atria are the filling stations of the heart; the ventricles are the pumping stations. The right ventricle pumps blood to the lungs for life-giving oxygen. The left ventricle pumps blood to the rest of the body.

How the Heart Works

The heart works like a double pump. The blood flows from the right atrium down to the right ventricle. This blood then goes out to the lungs. After the blood has been oxygenated in the lungs, it

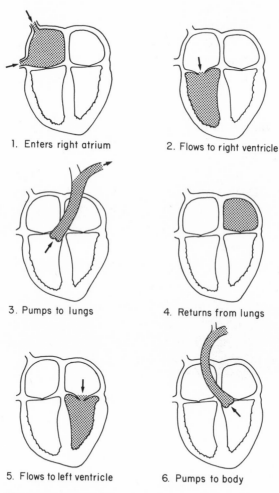

1. Enters right atrium   2. Flows to right ventricle

3. Pumps to lungs   4. Returns from lungs

5. Flows to left ventricle   6. Pumps to body

PASSAGE OF BLOOD THROUGH THE HEART

It takes blood about ten to fifteen seconds to make a complete circuit around the cardiovascular system. In this time, the heart at rest beats ten to twenty times.

flows back to the left side of the heart. It goes into the left atrium, then down into the left ventricle and out to the body. It passes to the body through the largest blood vessel of all, the *aorta* or great artery.

Pumping blood to the entire body as the left ventricle does is a more difficult task and requires more work than just pumping to the lungs. Therefore, the left ventricle has a thicker wall than the right ventricle. It generates about five times as much pressure as the right ventricle. This is because each ventricle pumps the exact same amount of blood.

Both ventricles contract simultaneously. The flow to the lungs is exactly the same as the flow to the body. Otherwise, the body would have an imbalance in volume and could not function.

How the Heart Beats

How do the heart chambers know when to contract and when to relax. The heart is set into continuing motion by a network of nerve cells threaded throughout the heart but much too small to see.

These are centered in a tiny bundle of nerve tissue in the right atrium called the *sinoatrial node*. This is the heart's own spark plug. From this bit of nerve tissue, an electric wave starts across the atria like a ripple across a pond. In the wake of this wave of electric energy, the atria contract forcing blood down into the ventricles. Part of the electric wave then travels swiftly down a connecting nerve between the atria and the ventricles, called the *atrioventricular node*. Below the atrioventricular node is a bundle of electrical connections that carry the contraction wave into the ventricles.

Most muscles in the body depend on a nerve connection to the brain. For example, if the nerves connecting the arm to the brain were cut, the arm would be paralyzed. But heart muscle is different. It needs no connection to the rest of the nervous system.

Valves: The Heart's Swinging Doors

The heart has valves to keep the blood flowing in the right direction. These valves function like the sails of a boat, ballooning when the pressure increases in the ventricle. When the valves balloon, the area between the ventricle and the atrium closes tightly.

When the pressure drops and the valve collapses, just as the sail collapses when the wind ceases, the valves open and blood flows from the atrium into the ventricle.

A valve is located between each atrium and ventricle. This valve opens downward into the ventricle. A valve is also located at the outlet from each ventricle. When the ventricles contract, these valves are forced open; the blood rushes into the pulmonary artery and the aorta. When the ventricles relax, the valves close, shutting off any backward flow into the ventricles. A famous cardiologist described heart valves as being "soft as silk and strong as steel."

What Goes Wrong

If the heart is so miraculous, what goes wrong? Interestingly, it is not the heart itself which usually fails. The problem involves the blood supply to the heart. When this supply is inadequate, the heart does not have the power to work properly. Then the heart runs into trouble.

Being a muscle, the heart requires blood. While the heart is busy pumping blood to all parts of the body, it must also constantly receive its own supply of blood. Because the heart works so incessantly (contracting more than 100,000 times a day), the heart has

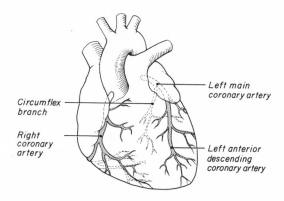

THE CORONARY ARTERIES

Pencil-thin, the coronary arteries are the only source of blood for the heart. (The heart cannot use the blood passing through its chambers.)

tremendous blood needs. This blood must reach the heart through the *coronary arteries*.

A Crown More Precious than Diamonds

The coronary arteries sit on top of the heart like a crown. These arteries are the *sole* blood supply to the heart. Any significant interference with the blood flow through these vessels affects the entire functioning of the heart.

With all the blood racing through the heart each minute, it seems impossible that the blood supply to the heart would not be sufficient. But the walls of the heart are watertight and blood cannot seep through to the layers of heart muscle. Blood is carried to the heart only through these coronary arteries.

The coronary arteries are end arteries. This means that each branch sends blood to one specific area of heart muscle. If this branch is blocked, the muscle that depends on it will die.

There are two principal coronary arteries. They are the right coronary artery and the left main coronary artery. The left main coronary artery divides into two branches: the left anterior descending artery and the left circumflex artery.

Each artery supplies a different area of the heart. Briefly, the left anterior descending artery supplies most of the front wall of the left ventricle, a portion of the interventricular septum as well as the front wall of the right ventricle. The left circumflex artery supplies the left side of the left ventricle and the left atrium. The right coronary artery supplies the right atrium and the right ventricle along with the posterior portions of the left ventricle and the interventricular septum.

PENCIL-THIN BUT POWERFUL

Coronary arteries are amazingly small considering their great importance. In a full-grown man, coronary arteries are about four or five inches in length and only one-eighth of an inch in diameter —slightly wider than the lead in a pencil.

When the heart is working hard, the flow through the coronary arteries can be as much as three pints per minute. Ordinarily about half a pint per minute passes through the coronary arteries. (The heart pumps about five to six quarts of blood a minute. About 5 percent of this returns through the coronary arteries to feed the heart muscle.) The reason the coronary arteries can carry this extraordinary blood flow is that they are not rigid. They dilate and widen in response to the heart's increased work load. This property is lost in diseased coronary arteries.

Anything that narrows the coronary arteries or interferes with their ability to expand can decrease the supply of blood to the heart. This will interfere with the heart's ability to function—at first under stress when the heart needs extra oxygen and blood, and later even under ordinary conditions.

Atherosclerosis: The Trouble Maker

Doctors say *atherosclerosis* is the main cause of coronary artery narrowing and thus heart attacks.

If the narrowing is severe enough to prevent adequate oxygen from reaching the heart muscle, atherosclerosis or coronary heart disease is said to exist. Normally coronary arteries are smooth and firm so blood can flow with a minimum of interference. Atherosclerosis makes the arteries rough and wrinkled.

The heaviest plaques of cholesterol are commonly found at places where the arteries are bent as much as 80 degrees. At these points, where the bend is almost at right angles, there is already a narrowing of the arterial passageway.

It is important to realize, however, that the critical factor is not the mere presence of these deposits but rather the extent of blood flow blockage. It is the total blood supply to the myocardium rather than the state of the arteries that determines whether the disease will be serious.

If the degree of obstruction is moderate and does not significantly reduce the blood to the heart, the disease may never be suspected. In fact, many men in the United States have evidence of some coronary atherosclerosis by age fifty; it is only the degree of involvement that varies.

Atherosclerosis can be categorized into four grades. Grade 1 atherosclerosis indicates the diameter of the artery is reduced by no more than 25 percent; Grade 2 represents a 50 percent reduction; Grade 3, a 75 percent reduction; and Grade 4, complete 100 percent

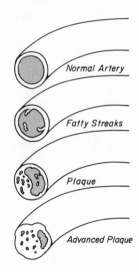

ATHEROSCLEROSIS

In coronary artery disease, not all coronary arteries are affected equally. Some may remain clear; others may have fatty deposits which narrow the blood vessels and decrease blood flow through these vessels.

obstruction. It is believed that an obstruction of at least 75 percent is necessary to produce a significant reduction in coronary blood flow; lesser degrees of narrowing can usually be tolerated without affecting heart function.

Until recently, there was no way (except at autopsy) to determine the degree of arterial obstruction or the arteries involved. But with *coronary arteriography,* a technique which permits the arteries to be visualized by X rays, it is now possible to identify the site and extent of atherosclerotic lesions with considerable accuracy. The procedure involves the insertion of a catheter into the aorta (by way of a peripheral artery) and the injection of a radio-iodine dye into the openings of the two main coronary arteries. As the dye is being injected a rapid series of X-ray films is taken to outline the arterial tree. Advanced atherosclerotic deposits can be easily detected in this way.

As you can see, your body is much like a car. If the gas line (coronary artery) is clogged, gasoline and air cannot get to the cylinders (the heart). Therefore the cylinders cannot pump properly. When this happens, a mechanic comes, blows out the fuel line and your engine starts up again. But with clogged coronaries it is not so easy. Medical science still does not know how to clear out congested coronary arteries. Surgeons can only bypass them and create a new path, thus the commonly done bypass operation.

DANGER SPOTS

Blockage can occur in any coronary artery. But it is more serious in certain arteries. The following are the most dangerous spots for a blockage to form.

1. The most dangerous is the main stem of the left coronary artery before it branches into its two main subdivisions. A total blockage in this area is rare. But when coronary arteriograms show a severe narrowing here, the patient is urged to have surgery immediately.
2. The second most deadly site is the left anterior artery before it branches off. Unfortunately, this is much more common. Dr. Donald Effler, the internationally known heart surgeon at the Cleveland Clinic, has aptly named this "The Widow Maker." Again, if severe narrowing is discovered without good collaterals, surgery is recommended.
3. The right coronary artery is another danger spot. This artery is wide to enable it to supply a large part of the bottom and back of the heart. Should it become significantly blocked, great damage could occur in these areas.
4. The circumflex branch of the left coronary artery is another danger point.

    The left ventricle can lose 20 to 25 percent of its muscle and still perform acceptably. However, if more than 25 percent of the left ventricle is destroyed, heart function may suffer.

    The heart's ability to relax is the first to weaken. The flow of blood from the lungs to the left ventricle can be slowed. The lungs become congested, and the person may have difficulty in breathing—the more heart muscle lost, the greater the breathing difficulty.

COLLATERALS CAN MAKE THE DIFFERENCE

Interestingly, the heart has its own bypass procedure. Sometimes the heart develops vessels to take the blood around the clogged arteries to the heart muscle. This is called *collateral circulation*.

It is of great importance since this network can often maintain an adequate blood supply to portions of the myocardium despite the presence of advanced atherosclerosis.

As people grow older, there is more time for cholesterol deposits to accumulate. But there is also more time for collateral vessels to develop. This is one reason why some younger men who have heart attacks often do not recover as readily as older men who have lived long enough to establish adequate collateral circulation. Interestingly, some theories now suggest that exercise aids in the development of collateral vessels.

Angina: A Warning

Atherosclerosis, by definition, means that the heart is not getting enough blood. The most common symptom of this problem is chest pain, or *angina pectoris*.

Where Is the Pain? Someone with angina rarely points to his chest with a finger or two. Instead, the person is likely to place a clenched fist, an entire open hand or both hands or fists against the chest in describing the pain.

Pain is usually under the breastbone. It may radiate to the left or right arm, the neck, the jaw, the teeth, or the upper back.

How Does It Feel? "It's not really a pain—it's more like a pressure or tightness," one victim explained. The severe pressure compels you to stop whatever you are doing. It is frightening as well as painful. This frightening aspect is another hallmark of angina.

How Long Does It Last? Angina is characteristically short. It lasts only seconds to a minute or a few minutes. It should not last twenty minutes, for example. The pain is steady and is not influenced by change in body position or breath-holding. Long-lasting chest pain (over ten minutes) may indicate a heart attack.

What Causes Angina? Any condition that increases the heart's demand for oxygen can cause angina. In general, oxygen demand is related to the amount of work the heart does.

As you would imagine, angina is usually brought on by physical effort. Conversely, angina is relieved by rest. When the activity stops, the oxygen demand decreases and the pain subsides. In addition, emotional stress may cause the heart to work harder and angina may result.

Can It Be Cured? Each episode of angina can be totally cured. One of the things that distinguishes angina from a heart attack is there is no permanent damage to the heart, but angina does tend to recur.

Nitroglycerin relieves angina. It works within a minute or two. If nitroglycerin is not effective, a more serious attack might be suspected and a doctor should be contacted immediately. Nitroglycerin acts by decreasing venous return to the heart and possibly by dilating the coronary vessels, thus decreasing the work load on the heart and increasing the blood flow and oxygen supply to the heart. Taken before stress situations, it can also prevent anginal episodes.

Stable and Unstable Angina. In most cases, angina is predictable. It occurs with certain types of physical effort or emotional stress, and it is relieved promptly by rest or nitroglycerin. This is called *stable angina.* However, if the pain pattern suddenly worsens and becomes unpredictable, occurring spontaneously or at rest, and is no longer controlled consistently by nitroglycerin, the condition is termed *unstable angina.* Unstable angina generally indicates progression of coronary disease and is more serious than stable angina.

Be aware:

Chest pains can stem from many things—some have nothing to do with the heart. If you suspect angina but can't be certain, don't feel stupid. Only a physician can make a diagnosis of angina.

A person who has had angina may not realize a heart attack is occurring. He may assume it is angina again. Typically, the pain that occurs with a heart attack may last for hours and does not subside until a narcotic such as morphine is administered.

If there is any question, seek help *immediately.*

Heart Attack!

If there is a sustained lack of oxygen to a section of heart muscle, the cells in that area cannot live. Local tissue death occurs. This is a heart attack, or *acute myocardial infarction*.

A heart attack is usually due to a sudden blockage of an already narrowed coronary artery. The exact reason a sudden blockage occurs is not completely understood. Three different causes have been suggested:

POSSIBLE CAUSE #1:

A blood clot may develop on the roughened surface of an atherosclerotic plaque. The blood, flowing through a roughened artery, may receive a trouble signal to clot. Similarly, a cut finger sends out a trouble signal, and a clot forms to protect us from bleeding.

POSSIBLE CAUSE #2:

The atherosclerotic deposit may damage the underlying arterial wall and cause bleeding beneath the plaque. This subintimal

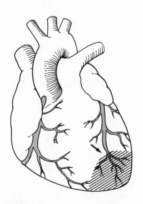

A HEART ATTACK

The shaded area depicts a typical heart attack. This part of the heart muscle has died due to inadequate blood supply (note the narrowed arteries). Despite such damage, the heart can continue functioning well for many years.

hemorrhage may dislodge the plaque which then obstructs the vessel.

POSSIBLE CAUSE #3:

A piece of large plaque may break off, move along and block a smaller artery.

Although these possible causes offer a logical explanation for this sudden event, it is now clear that they cannot account for *all* heart attacks. Autopsies have shown that some heart attacks develop even though the coronary arteries are not blocked, and a heart attack may occur even with normal coronary arteries. In these cases, the heart may have an enormous demand for oxygen at a particular moment (for example, during vigorous exercise or shoveling snow). This demand cannot be met by the available blood supply. Even though the arteries are not blocked, the heart's demand for oxygen simply overwhelms the supply and some heart tissue dies from lack of oxygen. This is the most commonly accepted explanation for this puzzling occurrence.

Cardiac Crisis

Many heart-attack victims never reach the hospital; about 400,000 die each year before getting there, as many as 60 percent in the first hour. Yet, damage to the heart muscle is rarely enough to cause death. What is lethal is the disruption in the electric spark initiating heart-muscle contraction. This disruption may be due to the sudden changes in rhythm due to the heart attack.

Fibrillation Alert

The most dangerous rhythmic disorder is *ventricular fibrillation*. This means the lower chambers of the heart contract in an uncoordinated manner, causing blood pumping to cease completely. Treated within one minute the patient has a 90 percent or better chance of surviving. A delay of four minutes means a survival rate of less than 10 percent because of extensive and irreversible brain and heart damage.

Fibrillation can be cured, but it must be done immediately. Doctors use an instrument called a *defibrillator*, a plate applied to the chest. A jolt of electricity is passed through the defibrillator into the heart muscle to get the heart back on the right tempo.

Even better, it is now possible to prevent ventricular fibrillation, so that the heart will not have to tolerate even brief episodes of this arrhythmia. Ventricular fibrillation may be heralded by an early warning sign—an identifiable disturbance in the heartbeat—that can be picked up by the coronary care monitoring equipment. The staff immediately gives heart-calming medicines including lidocaine. In this way, danger is avoided.

Coronary care units are remarkably effective. These units have reduced heart attack deaths among hospitalized patients up to 30 percent. If all heart attack victims could receive such care in the first few hours, more than 50,000 lives could be saved each year!

Assessing Your Attack

Most heart attacks damage the main pumping chamber, the left ventricle (right ventricular heart attacks are rare), not the whole ventricle but just a portion. The damage depends primarily on which vessel is blocked; this determines the area of the heart which is affected.

The seriousness of a heart attack depends on the specific area of the heart involved even more than the size of the area destroyed. A small heart attack affecting a vital area can be much more dangerous than a large one that spares such portions of the organ.

Doctors consider location as one factor in explaining the prognosis because complications vary according to the affected area. Heart attacks in the front or anterior wall tend to have a higher death rate than those that affect the lower or inferior portion. Potentially fatal abnormalities affecting the electrical system also vary according to the location of the heart attack.

To define the areas affected, doctors use specific medical terms. These include:

1. *Anterior infarction.* When the left coronary artery or its branches are blocked and the front (anterior) heart wall is affected.

2. *Inferior infarction.* When the right coronary artery is blocked and the bottom (inferior) wall of the left ventricle is affected.

3. *Anterolateral infarction.* When the damage involves both the front and the left outside walls of the left ventricle.

4. *Anteroseptal infarction.* When there is damage to both the front wall and the interventricular septum.

5. *Subendocardial infarction.* Damage to only the inside part of the ventricular wall—that wall next to the inner lining or endocardium.

6. *Transmural.* Widespread damage extending through the entire ventricular wall (from the endocardium to the epicardium). This is usually the most serious, especially in the early recovery period.

Showing Off Your Scar

People always love to show off their scars as evidence of a battle fought and won. There is a definite scar after a heart attack, but it can be seen only on electrocardiagram tracings.

However, the scar is extremely significant. It can determine life or death immediately after a heart attack. The scar has three zones. The first zone contains the tissue damaged beyond repair. Surrounding this dead tissue is a second zone of heart cells which, although injured, are still able to survive if adequate circulation to the area is restored. Zone 3 is called the zone of ischemia. This contains cells that can be expected to recover unless the heart damage worsens. So the ultimate damage depends on how Zone 2 and Zone 3 fare.

The Beat Goes On

The heart sounds complex and fragile; actually it is remarkably strong. Many people imagine the heart must be in perfect condition, but, in fact, nature compensates. When, for example, one of the auricles is unable to contract, the ventricle simply takes over and fills itself. If similarly, the valvular opening between the auricle and ventricle is partially damaged, the auricle just pumps harder to force blood through the narrowed opening. Indeed, there have been cases where over 60 percent of the left ventricle was completely dead—yet the remaining muscle successfully pumped blood to the rest of the body.

9. Your Risk Checklist

AFTER a first heart attack, most people are terrified they will have another one. It is important to realize that one heart attack does not doom a person to a second heart attack.

"I feel great—even better than before my attack," one man told us. No one is actually better than before; damage to the heart cannot be undone. However, a healthier life style can be pursued. This means reducing your risk factors—the elements which contribute to the development of heart attacks. No one factor alone is responsible. The more risk factors you have, the deeper in the "Danger, watch out!" area you are. To estimate your chances of having a heart attack, take this simple test:

Test Yourself

1. Are you male and past forty?
   Yes ___   No ___
2. Do you have a family history of heart attacks at an early age?
   Yes ___   No ___
3. Do you smoke?
   Yes ___   No ___
4. Do you have high blood pressure?
   Yes ___   No ___
5. Are you under stress and tension in your daily life?
   Yes ___   No ___
6. Are you overweight?
   Yes ___   No ___
7. Do you have high levels of cholesterol and other fats in your blood?
   Yes ___   No ___

8. Do you have diabetes or gout?

Yes ___ No ___

9. Do you lead a sedentary life?

Yes ___ No ___

10. Do you have an overly ambitious, competitive, aggressive, impatient personality?

Yes ___ No ___

The Risk Factors Explained

Ten years ago, doctors knew little about risk factors. Today, they can pinpoint the risks, and, more importantly, they can tell you how to avoid them.

Most risk factors (eight out of ten) can be changed, and altering just one factor may significantly cut your risk because the factors interact. For example, are you overweight? Simply by reducing your weight, you will also probably lower your blood pressure, lower your cholesterol, lessen your risk of diabetes, and perhaps increase your physical activity level.

After decades of increasing death rates from heart attacks, a dramatic decline in death has occurred between 1968 and 1976. While the causes are numerous—more coronary care units, better drugs, more mobile coronary units—it is believed that changes in the identifiable risk factors do account for much of this decline.

Today, people seem more weight conscious. Older people have begun to exercise in their leisure time. Mothers no longer believe that a fat baby is a healthy baby. Low fat milk and margarine products are an accepted way of eating. And everyone recognizes the effect of our emotions on our physical health.

To understand how risk factors contribute to heart disease, let's examine each factor more closely.

Male and Past Forty

Heart attacks are much more common in men than women. About 600,000 people die of heart attacks each year—400,000 are men, 200,000 are women.

During the childbearing years women are seemingly protected by their hormones. After menopause, however, the rate of heart attacks in women rises precipitously and eventually equals the rate in men.

In both men and women, the greater the age, the greater the risk. For example, a man in his fifties has four times the risk of a heart attack as a man in his thirties. Unfortunately, heart attacks can and do occur in men as young as thirty and sometimes even younger.

While women are less likely to have attacks, studies show they do not recover as quickly. Dr. Melvin J. Stern, associate clinical professor of psychiatry at George Washington University Medical Center in Washington, D.C., did studies comparing the recovery in men and women. More than half of the patients who did poorly, he found, were women.

"These women were reduced to people who had no status and invariably they became depressed," noted Dr. Stern. Unmarried women did the poorest. Drugs can help depression after a heart attack. But Dr. Stern stressed that women who survive heart attacks should resume activities as much as possible and get professional counseling if symptoms of depression persist.

A Family History of Heart Attacks at an Early Age

Heredity certainly ranks high among the risk factors. This is particularly true if a father or grandfather died in his forties or fifties of a heart attack. Studies have found that a man's father, grandfather, and brothers will often develop a heart attack at the same age. It has been postulated (but not proved) that the physical structure of the coronary arteries and the rate of atherosclerosis may be genetically determined.

Are you doomed by your inheritance? Not necessarily. Doctors say it is *not* simply a matter of genes. It may be a matter of lifestyle. For example, a person may have an inherited tendency to be overweight, but he may *be* overweight due to poor eating habits.

A child with two thin parents has an 8 percent chance of being obese; a child with one obese parent has a 44 percent chance; a child with two obese parents has an 88 percent chance of being overweight. Bad genes? Possibly. But orphans and children with foster parents generally follow the same pattern as their adoptive, not their biological, parents.

Exercise is still another component of your lifestyle. Surveys show that parents who exercise are more likely to have children who exercise. Children are even likely to select the same sport.

By changing environmental factors—diet, smoking, weight, high blood pressure, and stress that may have affected family members in the past—doctors believe you can lessen your hereditary risk.

Smoking

The risk of a heart attack is nearly double in cigarette smokers. A single cigarette can speed up heartbeat, increase blood pressure, and alter blood flow. According to a study done in Israel, smoking also lowers the level of high-density lipoproteins which have a protective effect against atherosclerosis. (Smoking cigars or a pipe presents less risk.)

"I realize that no fully sane individual smokes because he thinks it's healthy," admitted a heart patient. "I'd like to stop if I could, but there's a fire at both ends of every cigarette. The fire in me forces me to light the match to the other end of that cigarette."

Quitting is tough, but behavioral scientists believe smoking is a habit, not an addiction. Understanding the dangers of smoking is important.

When a smoker inhales his favorite cigarette, he accumulates carbon monoxide in his blood. Hemoglobin has an affinity for carbon monoxide and mixes with it. Hemoglobin's affinity for carbon monoxide is 200 times greater than its affinity for oxygen. So only a tiny amount of carbon monoxide is needed to displace oxygen from the hemoglobin. Inadequate oxygen can cause angina.

Unfortunately, people who switch to non-nicotine cigarettes still have this problem. A West Coast doctor tested his patients with nicotine and non-nicotine cigarettes and found no difference in the effect on the smoker's electrocardiogram or stress tests.

Smoking can produce changes in the electrocardiogram. "We ask our patients not to smoke for at least twelve hours before they come for an exercise EKG," stated one cardiologist.

Smokers also have a tendency to develop irregular heartbeats, which may increase the danger of sudden death. Smokers of two packs of cigarettes a day have an incidence of sudden death from heart attacks five times greater than those of nonsmokers. The latest figures show that the death rate from coronary heart disease is 70 percent higher for men smokers; it is 50 percent higher for women smokers.

Cigarettes are troublemakers not only for the person smoking but for others exposed to "secondhand smoke." Bernard Ecadow, Ph.D. and Martin I. Blake, pharmacists at the University of Illinois, have shown that tiny particles—less than a millionth of a meter in diameter—can cling to lung surfaces and be dangerous for those with heart problems. So most doctors recommend heart patients avoid smoky rooms for extended periods of time.

High Blood Pressure

High blood pressure sharply increases the chances of a heart attack. A man whose blood pressure at systole is higher than 160 has four times the risk of a person with systolic under 120.

Blood pressure is recorded as a fraction, for example 130/80. The first figure is the systolic, the pressure when the heart pumps; the second is the diastolic, the pressure between beats. Blood pressure is a measure of the force against the walls of the arteries. Each time the heart pumps blood, your pressure increases; in the interval between beats, the pressure goes down.

What constitutes high blood pressure varies somewhat with age but in general, repeated readings that stay about 140/100 are considered cause for concern in a person who is young or middle-aged.

You may have high blood pressure and not know it. Twenty million Americans—10 percent of the population—have high blood pressure and most are totally unaware of it. Hypertension is often called "the silent killer" because it produces no symptoms. But it does kill—the average life expectancy of a person with untreated high blood pressure is fifty-two years.

The longer hypertension is left untreated, the greater the likelihood the heart will be affected. So it is imperative to have your blood pressure checked once a year.

A few people—about 15 percent of all hypertensives—have *secondary hypertension*. This means the cause can be identified. It is sometimes an obstruction of blood flow to the kidney due to atherosclerotic deposits. This is occasionally improved through surgery.

Unfortunately, most people (85 percent of all hypertensives) have *essential hypertension*. This means no simple cause can be found. However, essential hypertension can almost always be controlled.

Essential hypertension usually first occurs when a person is in his thirties. One widely accepted theory states that hypertension may occur only occasionally at first, usually during periods of stress.

Repeated episodes affect pressure-sensitive cells called baroreceptors. Situated in strategic places along the arterial system, these centers are thought to be reset to help maintain normal blood pressure, just as a thermostat works to keep a house at a preset temperature. Exposure to recurrent elevated blood pressure episodes may bring about a resetting of the baroreceptors—or barostats—to a new higher normal. Once reset, the barostats may sustain hypertension.

Too Good to Give Up

Fascinating new studies seem to suggest that some people learn unconsciously to raise their blood pressure because the higher pressure relieves the pains and anxieties of life.

Support for this hypothesis was found recently in experiments with rats at the New York Hospital, Cornell Medical Center, in New York City. The experiments showed that the animals with high blood pressure were slower to avoid a painful stimulus than rats whose pressure was normal. The difference appeared to lie simply in the animals' perception of discomfort. The "noxious stimuli" evidently seemed less intense or less important to the animals when their blood pressure was high.

This new hypothesis suggests that animals and humans can be taught to change their blood pressure. It is hoped that people who control stress this way can be identified and then trained to find other strategies for dealing with unpleasant pressure-raising experiences.

Interestingly, certain people are more prone to high blood pressure than others. Better educated people are less likely to have high blood pressure. In women, pressure is generally lower than in men until about age fifty, after which the situation is reversed. Body size also appears to influence blood pressure. According to leading studies, the smaller the body, the lower the blood pressure.

Daily Stress and Tension

"Don't get excited or you'll have a heart attack." This warning is common. Heart attacks at moments of sudden stress are well known. There are cases of men who experience heart attacks when playing golf, or when gambling at cards, or when having an argument. For years, people believed sudden stress caused heart attacks. Today, doctors believe stress aggravates an already existing condition. And they say the dangerous type of stress is not sudden stress but *prolonged* stress.

How can stress affect the heart? When we become tense or anxious or angry, the brain sends out signals that cause physical changes. One of these changes is a constriction of the small arteries known as "arterioles." When the arterioles contract, it takes more pressure to pump blood through them. Since we know this contraction happens in the arterioles, doctors believe it also happens in the coronary arteries. If the coronary arteries are partially clogged with fatty deposits, constriction could result in a blockage.

What is too much stress? Psychologist Frances Meritt Stern, director of the Institute for Behavioral Awareness in Springfield, New Jersey, has developed a stress quiz designed to help you evaluate your on-the-job stress level.* A short version of this stress quiz follows. Complete it, then score yourself.

To score, write 1 (for the least), 2, or 3 (the most) for each

* Reprinted by permission of the Institute for Behavior Awareness, Springfield, New Jersey.

of the twenty statements. In deciding on the number of points, consider how strongly or intensely you experience discomfort on the job, and how often these situations arise. For example, an intense stressor that occurs often would receive a three rating. A stressor that is fairly strong and/or happens some of the time would be rated a two. A stressor that occurs rarely and/or is not very strong would be rated a one.

1. I lose sleep over work-related problems.
2. I think I'm worth more than my paycheck shows.
3. I dread being evaluated by a superior or boss.
4. I worry about dealing with deadlines that can't be met.
5. I'm afraid others' expectations of me in my present job are unclear.
6. It's difficult for me to criticize another's work.
7. I don't feel good about myself because of my job.
8. It's frustrating not being part of decision-making that alters the scope of my job.
9. My back and/or neck tense while I'm working.
10. I feel uncomfortable having to work closely with people I find it hard to get along with.
11. I have difficulty dealing with my supervisory responsibilities.
12. I feel under a lot of pressure at work.
13. My stomach ties in knots at work.
14. I think about finding another job.
15. My body becomes tense while I'm working.
16. I believe there is not enough time to get everything done.
17. I feel my work is causing me head pain.
18. It's upsetting having to deal with unrealistic demands made by a supervisor or boss.
19. I don't like having to do things I know are wrong.
20. I don't believe my work is appreciated by my superiors.

SCORING INFORMATION

Total the number of points. A score of 31–49 can be considered the mid-range. Toward the upper limits of that range, you may be beginning to experience more tension than is healthy. A score of 50–60 would denote very high stress and an unhealthy situation. Evaluating the source of the stress may help eliminate it. A high score on statements 9, 13, 15, and 17 shows too much body stress. A high score on 1, 2, 3, 4, 7, 12, 14, 16, and 20 shows needless destructive worry. A high score on 3, 5, 6, 8, 10, 11, 18, and 19 shows stress related to inability to get along with others.

Most laymen rate stress higher in the list of risk factors than medical studies actually warrant. All the same, stress *is* important because it increases the likelihood of three other risk factors. A person's blood pressure will rise in stressful situations, smoking is more likely, and evidence even points to increases in serum cholesterol.

Overweight

Extra pounds make the heart work harder—every minute of every day. As one saying goes, "Your fat is your fate." The American Heart Association puts it even more bluntly, "Pity the fat man, the statisticians number his days." The Framingham Study has shown that men who are 30 percent overweight have almost a three-times-greater risk of developing heart disease than those who were 10 percent or more underweight.

Why is excess weight so bad? For one thing, excess weight increases the likelihood of high blood pressure. It also increases the risk of blood lipid abnormalities and diabetes.

Being overweight is a national problem. Unfortunately, over half of all Americans are overweight. Reducing and keeping weight off is not easy, but understanding caloric needs will help you plan a sensible eating regime.

Your doctor will probably give you a diet and help you plan your total caloric needs. But there is a simple rule-of-thumb in estimating your daily diet. Generally, it takes about 15 calories a day to maintain a pound of body weight. So if you weigh 150 pounds, you need 2,250 calories a day to maintain your present weight. If you want to reduce at the rate of a pound a week, you must cut down by 500 calories a day. You can cut 150 calories each day by taking a half hour walk a day. Therefore, you should eliminate 350 calories of food to provide a daily diet of 1,900 calories. Ways to cut these calories are discussed later in this book.

High Levels of Cholesterol and Other Fats in the Blood

The following case history is true:

A fifty-year-old man entered the emergency room complaining of severe pain in his stomach, which had begun abruptly that morning. X rays showed probable evidence of an abdominal aortic aneurysm, a weakening in the wall of the main blood vessel of the abdomen. As the X ray was being read, the patient went into shock. He was rushed to the operating room and a Dacron graft was inserted in the blood vessel. The patient survived the operation but died two weeks later of complications secondary to the shock and surgery.

Before the sudden onset of his illness, this man had been vigorous and active with no symptoms of any heart or vascular disease. An aneurysm is usually caused by deposits in the blood vessel, which weaken it and eventually lead to a rupture of the blood vessel wall. Cholesterol is a major component of these deposits.

Many studies have shown an association between the levels of cholesterol and other blood fats and heart attacks. The Framingham Study, for example, has found that the frequency of coronary heart disease is seven times greater in persons with cholesterol values above 259 than among those with values below 200.

Cholesterol, one of the fatty materials found in the blood, is not all bad. Indeed, it is a necessary part of every cell of the body. Scientists believe it may play a role in regulating the passage of nutrients into and out of the cells through the cell membranes. There is a high concentration of cholesterol in the brain. (That's why cardiologists may tell you not to eat brains or other organ food. It is also the reason pediatricians do not want very young children placed on low cholesterol diets.) But too much cholesterol can be dangerous.

It is important to note that high triglyceride levels also increase the risk of heart attack. Triglycerides come predominantly from the breakdown of starches (grains), carbohydrates, and some fatty substances. The Framingham Study, as well as others, found that even if the cholesterol level was moderate or low, the risk increased as the triglyceride level increased. Furthermore, people with high levels of both cholesterol and triglycerides seem to be worse off than those with high levels of one or the other.

There may be yet another very important factor in this picture: lipoproteins. Lipoproteins carry cholesterol from the liver to cells of the body; other lipoproteins remove unneeded cholesterol from body tissues and return it to the liver for excretion from the body. Low-density proteins (or LDL) are linked to high risk of clogging and heart disease. On the other hand, high-density proteins (HDL) may possibly reduce the risk of clogging. Doctors can now do simple blood tests to determine whether the dangerous LDLs or the protective HDLs are active in the body.

Diabetes or Gout

Heart attacks develop more frequently and earlier in people with diabetes. Researchers have found that cholesterol tends to be higher in diabetics than in non-diabetics. High blood pressure is nearly twice as frequent, and four out of every five diabetics are overweight. For these reasons, diabetics are more prone to multiple heart attacks in early to mid-adult life. The Framingham Study has found that the risk of death from heart disease is 2.3 times higher in diabetic men and 5.7 times higher in diabetic women.

Diabetes mellitus is a disorder of sugar metabolism. Sugar and starch that has been converted to sugar must be changed into energy in the cells. When there is not enough insulin, the body cannot turn sugar into energy properly. Sugar accumulates in the blood and spills over into the urine. Fatty substances also increase in the blood. These may be deposited in the blood vessel walls, causing atherosclerosis and possibly a heart attack.

Today the American Diabetes Association states that tight control of diabetes, careful attention to maintaining blood glucose at normal levels, and weight reduction may lessen the risk of a heart attack.

Gout, a disease caused by high uric acid levels in the blood, also increases the risk of having a heart attack.

"My mother has gout," a young mother told us. "She's a real stoic. This is the first time she really ever complained. And, you know, heart disease is in her family. Her brother had three attacks and her sister has had one."

Interestingly, gout is more common in men. The average victim is a middle-aged, overweight male who eats rich foods—also the typical heart attack victim.

Gout is very painful. An attack usually occurs during the night, often lodging in the big toe, but gout can also affect hands and fingers. Often the skin over the inflamed joint will scale or flake. (High blood uric acid levels may be present without pain. Your doctor can tell you if you have a "silent" elevation of uric acid.)

"How long will this terrible pain last?" the woman asked her doctor.

"Usually, gout lasts several hours or a day or two. But believe me, it's painful," the doctor answered.

"Isn't there something I can do for it?" she wondered.

"First of all, rest," he told her. "Then I'm going to give you a prescription for colchicine. This should relieve the pain. I am also going to prescribe allopurinol. This drug lowers uric acid and should decrease the frequency of your attacks." (Some doctors prescribe indomethasone which is very effective.)

The higher occurrence of heart attacks in people with diabetes and gout has led some scientists to theorize that a biochemical disturbance may cause heart attacks. This theory is now being investigated.

A Sedentary Life

Sedentary living—lack of physical activity—can increase one's risk of having a heart attack. It is now suspected that physical activity may increase the high-density lipoproteins that may be so valuable in decreasing atherosclerosis. At Kent State University, a researcher studied forty-two men ages thirty-nine to sixty-three, all in sedentary occupations. For an hour a day, five days a week, for nine months, these men took an intensive physical-fitness program. In every man, blood cholesterol declined, with the largest decline in those who had the highest levels at the start of the program.

Other studies suggest that physical activity can help lower

high blood pressure. For example, researchers at the San Diego State College Exercise Laboratory placed twenty-three men with high blood pressure on a moderate exercise program for an hour twice a week. Before the program, the average blood pressure for the group was 159/105. After six months, it was 148/93.

Exercise may also build collateral circulation. It is believed by many scientists that exercise over an extended time provides a controlled stress that may lead to the development of collateral vessels. It is even possible that if collateral circulation is great enough, a heart attack may be prevented since the spare vessel would take over immediately. Collateral circulation theories have not been proved but are still being studied.

Exercise relieves pent-up emotion and inner stress. One married couple, for example, insisted their secret of happiness was their taking walks whenever they found themselves arguing. When the argument got hot, the husband and wife would leave the house promptly without a further word, each going a separate way. The walk sometimes lasted half an hour or an hour. When they returned, they felt relieved and happy enough to kiss and make up.

Type of Personality

David Gluck (his name has been changed) was a real patient. He suffered a massive heart attack at age forty-two. Probably, his Type A personality contributed to this coronary event.

His office chart looked like this:

PATIENT'S NAME: David Gluck
AGE: 52
OCCUPATION: Director of American Liquor Distributors, Inc.
EDUCATION: Graduate, Harvard College; Harvard Business School; Ph.D. Economics, Wharton School
FAMILY HISTORY: Separated, father of three
PERSONALITY TRAITS: Fiercely ambitious, driving, always working against deadlines, highly competitive, a workaholic
PROBLEM: A first heart attack at age 42.

John T. Biggs, M.D., a St. Louis psychiatrist has pointed out that "The typical coronary-prone behavior includes competitiveness, aggressiveness, impatience, restlessness, explosive speech, sleeplessness, and constant haste. In addition to these symptoms, you may notice extra drinking and smoking and a possible mid-life crisis that blames everything on a wife and children."

Some years ago, a distinguished investigator observed that the coronary-prone individual is like the mythological Sisyphus, who passed the time in Hades pushing a large rock up a steep hill and never quite getting it there.

Recently, the affect of personality and behavior on the heart has been emphasized. Researchers believe there are two major personality types, Types A and B, with Type A being the coronary prone.

The Type A person is aggressive, ambitious, and competitive, has intense drive, must get things done and has little time to "waste" on the beauties of life such as travel, literature, art, and vacations. Type A's are often impatient, sometimes hostile. They try to finish every task as soon as possible, want to do everything by themselves, and will tackle increasingly larger work loads which are frequently beyond their capacity.

Type B personalities, on the other hand, are more easygoing, don't feel driven by time, and can enjoy leisure. Most of us are mixtures, but usually one or the other predominates in varying degrees.

One San Francisco study had laymen identify male friends who seemed typically Type A or Type B. Of the eighty-three men chosen as typical Type A's, twenty-three (28 percent) showed symptoms of heart disease. In contrast, only three of eighty-three Type B men showed evidence of heart disease.

A similar study was done for women. Of the Type A women (mainly women in industry or professional jobs), 19 percent showed heart disease, whereas only 4 percent of the Type B women (mainly housewives) had heart disease.

How can personality patterns affect the heart? One possible explanation is that stress causes cholesterol levels to rise. Another explanation is that stress causes abnormal amounts of adrenalin to be produced in the body. Adrenalin constricts blood vessels and raises blood pressure; it also affects the heart's demand for oxygen. Adrenalin can also cause irregularities of heartbeat (arrhythmias) which can be dangerous in the person with heart disease. Adrenalin may also make the blood platelets (participants in clotting) more sticky.

"You know the best way to live a long, long life?" an elderly surgeon asked us rhetorically. "Get a chronic disease and take care of it! It's the healthy ones that die young and suddenly!" Undoubtedly, taking care of heart disease makes an immense difference.

Many of us have atherosclerosis in one degree or another. It does not just occur in older people as was formerly believed. To prevent atherosclerosis from becoming a dangerous condition, we must understand its causes and then avoid these pitfalls.

10. Avoiding Another Attack

"IT's up to you," Dr. Rubenstein tells his patients. "Only you can reduce your own chances of having another heart attack." What Dr. Rubenstein is referring to is changing your lifestyle—eating patterns, exercise, and general life pace—so that you can reduce your risk of another heart attack.

Are people willing to make the necessary changes? "Most patients find it very difficult," Sheely McKeever, a medical assistant in a cardiologist's office, told us. "They are used to a certain lifestyle and pattern to their lives. They have been living a certain way for forty or fifty years and they are reluctant to change. Those who do change, change drastically. They try to live a totally healthy, completely new way."

Change is difficult for everyone. "For men, it seems particularly tough," Mrs. McKeever explained. "Women seem to change easier than men. Women are always on diets. They change jobs easily. For a man, it's much more difficult. They are extremely sensitive about losing their ability to provide for their families. A woman will come in and say she has to go on disability and she will smile. A man whispers it so no one else can hear and he's depressed about it."

"Should we move to Florida?" "Would it be better to leave the city?" people often ask. The role of climate is not totally understood, but doctors believe it is relatively unimportant. Hot, humid climates should be avoided since they can tax a weak heart. Is city living, with all its polluted air, harmful to the heart? At present, there is no convincing evidence that pollution is an important factor in heart disease. It should be added here that cigarette smoke contains much higher concentrations of pollutants than any city air.

Luckily, almost all the risk factors are controllable.

Controllable Risk Factors	Uncontrollable Risk Factors
Cigarette smoking	Heredity
High blood pressure	Male sex
Obesity	Age
High levels of cholesterol and other fats in the blood	
Diabetes or gout	
Sedentary lifestyle	
Type A personality	

To see how these factors can be controlled, let's examine each one.

Kicking the Smoking Habit

"I smoked for thirty-four years," said a fifty-three-year-old woman who had suffered one heart attack at age forty-eight and just undergone bypass surgery. "How did I stop? Very simple. The doctor scared me to death."

Like most habits, smoking is easier started than stopped, but quitting can make an immense difference. The Framingham Study found that heavy smokers who gave up smoking have, after several years, about the same incidence of heart attacks as people who never smoked. The American Cancer Society has stated: "Death rates from all causes rise with the number of cigarettes smoked daily."

Quitting has a strong initial success—usually 70 to 80 percent. The problem is, a year or so later the number usually drops to around 20 percent. Experts say if you can stop smoking completely for a month, chances are you will be an ex-smoker forever.

Here are some tips for giving up those dirty, expensive, and deadly cigarettes:

1. Change your brand to one you hate the most.
2. Ration yourself by counting out each morning the number you have decided to smoke. Place the rest out of easy reach.

3. Decrease your daily allowance.
4. Smoke each cigarette only halfway.
5. Get a friend or colleague to quit with you. Or join a local "smoke-ending" club.
6. Get up immediately after eating (a cigarette time for many).
7. Switch from coffee to some other beverage (this breaks the coffee/cigarette association).
8. Keep an unlighted cigarette around. Sometimes this satisfies the smoking urge.
9. Chew bits of fresh ginger. (Some find the taste is burning; others say it is cleansing and satisfying.)
10. Drink frequent glasses of water.
11. Nibble self-pleasing foods.
12. Skip familiar television programs, sit in a different comfortable chair, or stop reading the newspaper if these activities were associated with cigarette breaks.
13. Take deep breaths of air.
14. Buy yourself a present! If you have stopped a two-pack-a-day habit, you owe yourself a $10-a-week gift.
15. Exercise. You'll probably feel irritable and exercise will combat the feeling.

How to Lower Your Blood Pressure

For the person who has already had a heart attack, high blood pressure means more heart trouble may follow. So controlling high blood pressure is extremely important.

Thirty years ago, if you had high blood pressure, your doctor would tell you to lose weight, cut down on salt, and take a tranquillizer. If those things didn't work, you just had to pray.

Weight loss, salt restriction, and sedatives are still used (so is prayer!), but today high blood pressure *can* be controlled by drugs. If you are overweight, the best treatment is still dieting. Sometimes losing weight is all that is needed to control high blood pressure.

If these methods do not work, however, there are safe and highly effective drugs. In the 1980s, no one with high blood pressure should allow it to go untreated. Doctors usually begin by giving a diuretic or water pill. Because diuretics promote the removal of excess fluid from body tissues, blood pressure tends to fall toward normal.

If a diuretic alone is not adequate, other anti-hypertensive medicines may be given. Most likely, these will have to be taken for the rest of your life. However, most people get used to this routine without difficulty.

A Note: Nervousness can cause temporary high blood pressure. This is usually not serious, but temporary hypertension due to nervousness can sometimes be a forerunner of permanent high blood pressure.

Dizziness can occur with hypertensive drugs if a person stands up or bends suddenly. So, getting out of bed, rising from a chair, or bending from the waist should be done slowly.

Coping with Stress

Stress shows: People under stress look tense, they feel tense. They may shield their eyes, look away, or sit on the edge of their chair.

It is not the stress itself that destroys—it is how a person reacts to stress. "Fourteen hours of stress a day is not too much for a happy man but two hours may be too much for a disgruntled, insecure soul," a medical professor explained.

Dr. Marvin Belsky, a Manhattan internist makes this suggestion to his tense patients, "If a patient is really uptight I may ask him to close his eyes and imagine he's on a beach, remind him what the sand feels like under his feet, how the fresh air smells, what the waves sound like. It's not too difficult to train yourself to think of a pleasant experience that will relax and help free you for communication."

Another effective trick is proper, controlled breathing. When there is an abundance of oxygen in the body, muscles tend to relax. Since a tense person usually takes short breaths, his inhalation pattern actually inhibits relaxation. Taking slow deep breaths benefits the heart by providing a longer resting period between beats and thus reduces the heart's work load. Slow deep breathing also temporarily has a beneficial effect on high blood pressure.

Years ago, people believed the solution to stress was simply more time off. Interesting new studies have found that too little stress, a life devoid of challenges or changes, can produce many of the same symptoms and disorders as overwork. Indeed, the overwhelming majority of men answering a survey have indicated that they would continue to work, even if they suddenly became independently wealthy.

The answer to stress, therefore, seems to be in managing everyday pressures. This means working; it also means relaxing.

The following anti-stress tips were developed for corporate executives and their wives. But they apply to all workers—including housewives—as well.

10 Anti-Stress Tips

1. *Make a plan for each day.* List what you need to do. Begin by doing the most important tasks first. List only what you think you *can* accomplish rather than what you think you *should* accomplish.
2. *Avoid extra work.* Victims of stress should learn to say no. They must explain they have already overcommitted their time.
3. *Structure the day.* Whenever possible, set aside certain hours for phone calls, others for meetings, others for uninterrupted work.
4. *Allot time practically.* Decide how much time should realistically be spent on each project. Avoid getting bogged down with one task.
5. *Realize that human performance deteriorates after five hours.* Get into the habit of taking short breaks during the day. Stretch, do some deep breathing, or look out the window. You will get much more productivity out of your time once you have had a change of pace.
6. *Focus your total concentration on the task at hand.* Worrying about more than one thing at a time only dissipates energy.
7. *Approach work positively.* Remember the amount of work does not cause as much stress as the manner in which work is approached. Work at your own most comfortable pace.
8. *Delegate work.* Trying to do too many things—sometimes an impossible number at once—increases stress.

9. *Eliminate trivial tasks*. Delegate them or forget about them until a less busy time.

10. *Avoid wasting time*. Do not allow other people to waste your precious time. This means cutting off conversations quickly or closing the door to avoid unnecessary interruptions.

How to Slim Down

Overweight people know they are fat; they do not need to be told by a doctor. Many people who have been on the verge of losing weight for years find a heart attack triggers their "action button."

It would be simple to give an ideal diet here. Breakfast would account for x calories, lunch for y calories and dinner for whatever is left over. But the diet would be uninteresting, unappetizing, and no one would follow it.

So we are going to give some unorthodox suggestions. We hope they will make dieting a little easier and therefore a lot more successful.

Eat Your Favorite Foods, Nibble Often, and Other Strange Dieting Suggestions

Most doctors hand out a printed diet. Invariably, it does not contain the person's favorite food. Is it allowed? This depends, of course, on what else you eat. Let's take breakfast, for example.

Your Favorite Breakfast

½ cup coffee with cream and sugar	73 calories
1 glass juice	40 calories
Toast and butter	113 calories
2 eggs	146 calories
2 strips bacon	90 calories
TOTAL:	462 calories

You just love bacon, you say. You know it is high in fat and high in calories. Drearily, you conclude it must go but you're unhappy about it. Don't jump to conclusions. Here is a cardiologist-approved diet breakfast specially designed for you.

Your Doctor-Approved Breakfast

1 glass juice		40 calories
1 egg		73 calories
2 strips bacon		90 calories
Coffee (black)		0
	TOTAL:	203 calories

The idea is to individually adjust your diet to include your favorites. Cut out those items you enjoy less and modify others (coffee but no cream or sugar). Of course fatty foods such as bacon and high-cholesterol eggs should not be eaten every day, but they do not have to be avoided completely.

By carefully retaining your favorites, wherever possible, you will be a happier and more successful dieter. Ask for your doctor's help in reviewing your own plan. He will happily do it and probably will have other suggestions too.

NIBBLE AWAY

Unorthodox as it sounds, nibbling between meals might be just what you need. When you feel hungry, there are low concentrations of sugar in the blood. This increases your desire to eat. If you nibble at these times, it will not only provide sugar for the bloodstream, but also prevent you from overeating at mealtime. Parents tell their children not to eat before dinner because it kills their appetite. They are absolutely right—so nibbling (celery, carrots, toast without butter) is recommended.

EXERCISE BEFORE EATING

Many people think exercise makes you ravenous and you eat more. Actually, exercising before meals can kill the desire for food. The reasons are not known but scientists tell us that exercise before eating markedly reduces appetite.

SNIFF CHEAP PERFUME

Smell greatly alters appetite. We actually recognize foods by their odors, not tastes. If this process of smell association is interrupted, appetite is decreased. To do this, one doctor suggested smelling something just before a meal which you do not associate with eating. A few whiffs of cheap perfume kills even the most vigorous appetite.

How to Cut Your Cholesterol

Cutting calories is hard enough, but after a heart attack, fat and cholesterol must also be cut. In our country, almost everyone eats too much fat and cholesterol. In poorer countries where less animal fat is eaten, the incidence of heart attacks is much lower. It is appalling to realize that "normal" serum cholesterol levels in the U.S. are 200 to 240 whereas in countries where heart attacks are uncommon, normal cholesterol levels are only 100 to 120.

Here are some ways to lower cholesterol and fat intake.

The Essential Eight

1. Trim all visible fat from meat and poultry.
2. Use 2 percent fat skim milk rather than whole milk, liquid corn oil margarine rather than butter, liquid corn oil rather than hydrogenated oils.
3. Broil, roast, or bake meats and poultry instead of frying.
4. Use a roasting rack, a ribbed-bottom skillet, or ribbed broiler-pan. They enable fat to drip off the meats. Otherwise meats cook in their own drippings and the fat can be reabsorbed.
5. Eat beef, lamb, and pork only three times a week. The rest of the time, eat veal, chicken, and fish.
6. Avoid all commercial baked goods, creamy salad dressings, frostings, and glazings.
7. Don't eat the skin of chicken or turkey; avoid gravies.
8. Eat less generally and exercise more.

Be aware:

Some people with a hereditary predisposition for markedly elevated blood cholesterol and/or triglyceride levels may require more stringent regulation and even medication.

What Can Be Done about Diabetes and Gout?

Anybody can get diabetes. Thousands of people have it but are totally unaware of it. In the early stages or in mild cases, there may be no symptoms. Basically, diabetes tends to run in families and is discovered by a doctor through blood and urine tests. Most people who get diabetes are overweight. Diet alone is often enough to control diabetes and restore normal blood sugar levels in adults.

For years, doctors believed that controlling diabetes did not necessarily eliminate it as a risk factor in heart disease. Even with control, diabetes somehow seemed to contribute to the development of atherosclerosis. Recent evidence has shown that tight control of diabetes and careful attention to maintaining normal blood glucose levels can reduce the risk of heart disease.

Gout, a disease due to high uric acid levels in the blood, also contributes to heart attacks. Gout can usually be treated within twenty-four hours by an immensely effective drug called colchicine. A newer drug allopurinol acts by reducing production of uric acid. It also stimulates the breakdown and excretion of uric acid. If uric acid levels are abnormally high, whether or not gout attacks have occurred, doctors often prescribe a uric-acid-lowering drug.

Exercise Is Today's Edict

Today exercise is recommended almost from the first moment after a heart attack. Some commonly recommended exercise routines follow. *Remember, no exercise should be undertaken without consulting your doctor first.*

THE EARLY STAGE: *Just Home from the Hospital*
1. With arms on hips and legs slightly apart, rotate your trunk in all directions until you feel a bit of torso tightness.
2. Stretch neck backward and forward and side to side.
3. While lying on a double bed, roll over a couple of times to the left and then to the right for about a minute.
4. While lying on your back, tuck your knees gently up on your

chest and grab them with your arms (sort of like hugging yourself) then roll back and forth for a minute or so.

5. Take a short walk around the yard or down the block once a day.

THE MIDDLE STAGE: *Feeling Your Way*

On an empty bladder and an empty stomach, take a half hour stroll. Walk fifteen minutes in one direction (away from home) and then turn around and walk home.

After a while go fishing, play catch, ride a bike—do anything you have really missed during your temporary confinement.

FINAL STAGE: *Back to Normal*

If you have a favorite sport, you can probably return to it. Just relax and resume tasks in moderation. You can probably do things you may not have missed doing like housecleaning, trudging to the railroad station, and car washing.

Many people have questioned the significance of exercise, noting there were so many variables in exercise groups, it was inaccurate to single out exercise as a risk factor. But there is excellent evidence that a good exercise program *can* improve the heart's functioning and decrease angina.

Many scientists believe that regular exercise provides the kind of stress which promotes the development of collateral vessels. Some even believe that properly planned exercise may prolong life, although this point is not yet proven.

All exercise programs involve three basic principles:

EXERCISE PRINCIPLE #1: *Start slowly*. Don't strain or let your face become reddened.

EXERCISE PRINCIPLE #2: *Push yourself a little*. After you have become accustomed to a level of activity, try to go a little further.

EXERCISE PRINCIPLE #3: *Make it tougher*. As your strength and endurance increase, try to make your exercises gradually more strenuous.

Not everyone likes exercise. A fifty-year-old woman who had two heart attacks said she began exercising after her bypass surgery. "I started to exercise on a stationary bike for forty-five minutes a day. I despised every second." However, most people we spoke with found exercise enjoyable.

A warning:

An all-out sudden burst of activity after many years—even just many months—of relative inactivity can cause great aches and pain. It can also be lethal, placing sudden great strain on the heart. Consult your physician before exercising, and always exercise in moderation.

Slow Down: Your Type A Personality May Be Killing You

Most people who are Type A personalities are proud of it. The same characteristics which make them coronary prone—aggressiveness, drive, ambition, impatience—also make them successful. Dr. Irvine H. Page, a former heart attack victim himself, offers this tongue-in-cheek appraisal of the person with little risk:

He is an effeminate municipal worker or embalmer, completely lacking in physical and mental alertness, without drive, ambition, or competitive spirit, who has never attempted to meet a deadline at any time.

He is a man with poor appetite, subsisting on fruits and vegetables, laced with corn and whale oil, detesting tobacco, and spurning ownership of a TV, radio, or motor car. He has a full head of hair and is scrawny and unathletic in appearance, yet he is constantly straining his puny muscles by exercise.

He is low in income, blood pressure, blood sugar, uric acid, and cholesterol. He has been on nicotinic acid, pyridoxine, and anticoagulant therapy ever since his prophylactic castration.

Certainly this is an exaggeration but can a person really change his personality? A leading psychiatrist at Beth Israel Hospital in New York City told us, "It is not really possible for a person to change suddenly. You can tell them to act a certain way but they will only be able to play a part for so long."

What a person *can* do is set his life into a better rhythm. Type A's must learn how to act decisively when necessary and then to relax. This dynamic engagement and disengagement of the nervous system is really the only way to maintain a healthy mind and heart.

The key to success is realizing that relaxation is not a luxury: It is a necessity. Drs. Meyer Friedman and Roy Rosenman, developers of the Type A theory, have written a book entitled *Type A Behavior and Your Heart*. In it, they outline some steps to help Type A's relax. Some of their recommendations are:

1. Get up fifteen minutes earlier.
2. Analyze your work. Avoid the unnecessary.
3. Take more time for dinner and breakfast.
4. Realize what's important. "As you sweat over something," they say, "ask yourself if it's really going to make a difference in your life five years from now."
5. Concentrate on one thing at a time. "Remember," they write, "that even Einstein, when tying his shoelaces, thought chiefly about the bow. Don't let your mind wander. Concentrate on what you are doing at the moment."
7. Take short breaks. If you find that your work is inducing tension, take a break.
8. Avoid people who anger you.
9. Look well—this is somehow calming.
10. Make a conscious effort to spend one hour each day relaxing—read, play, or just daydream.

Making suggestions is easy, but following them in everyday life is very difficult. Dr. Rosenman, who has suffered two heart attacks, states strongly, "If you don't change your Type A behavior pattern, other protective measures against heart attack—a healthy diet, exercise, not smoking—may be largely a waste of time."

Try a Pet!

Changing lifelong patterns is difficult, but here's an easy (and happy) change—buy a pet! Believe it or not, people who own pets have an especially good chance of surviving the crucial first year after a heart attack.

Researchers from the University of Pennsylvania already knew that people who live alone are more likely to have heart disease, but they wanted to find out whether being alone also influenced recovery.

One measure of companionship—owning a pet—turned out to make a big difference. A study was done of ninety-two patients; fifty-three had pets and thirty-nine did not. Of the fifty-three who had pets only four died; of the thirty-nine without pets eleven died. Moreover, a pet made a difference regardless of how sick the person was.

Was it the affection or the exercise from walking the animal? This time the exercise advocates lost out. Researchers found that people who kept physically undemanding pets like cats, birds, gerbils, and lizards were still super-survivors.

So don't neglect "TLC." Tender Loving Care is still the best way to a happy heart and a healthy heart too.

II. Eating Less, Enjoying It More

A FIFTY-YEAR-OLD business executive: "You know what my favorite food is now? Bread! You know why? I'm starving!"

A forty-six-year-old salesman: "I've been overweight my whole life because I just love to eat. I really miss it."

A forty-eight-year-old building superintendent: "I was a real salter. At first, my wife made separate meals for me, but it was too much. Now we all eat the flat stuff and hate it."

A fifty-five-year-old lawyer: "You know what I miss most? Cheese. Every night my wife would serve cheese and cocktails. Funny, I don't miss the cocktails at all, but I really miss that cheese."

A forty-eight-year-old housekeeper: "I just love creamed corn and I can't have it. I really miss it, but I resist."

A sixty-year-old physician: "When I go to a restaurant, I never look at the menu. I just know. It's always the same . . . fish, broiled with no butter, and salad with no dressing, just pepper."

No one likes dieting, but everybody we spoke with admitted dieting made them feel better. "When I eat like a pig, I suffer. I feel loggy and tired as soon as I go off the diet," one man admitted.

Fat and Your Heart

Cardiologists have their favorite slogans. One tells patients, "The longer the belt, the shorter the life." Another warns, "You can dig your grave with your teeth." Unquestionably, they are right. For the person with a heart problem, extra pounds means trouble. Too much weight puts an added burden on the heart every minute, every day.

Middle-aged men who are 30 percent or more overweight run twice the risk of a heart attack compared to middle-aged men of normal weight.

Obesity can double or triple the risk of developing high blood pressure. The Framingham Heart Study, which monitored several thousand people, found that for each 10 percent excess in weight, blood pressure rose 6.5 mm. Conversely, lower weight is accompanied by an equivalent drop in blood pressure.

This has led some researchers to conclude that if all people were at their ideal weight, we'd have 25 percent less coronary heart disease and 35 percent less congestive heart failure.

Are You Too Fat?

Very likely you are. Obesity is the most common health problem in America today. Over 40 million of us—and the numbers are increasing—are simply too fat.

"It's my glands. I can't help it," many people say. The thyroid gland does play an important role in maintaining body weight, but overweight is rarely due to glandular imbalances or hypoglycemia. Only about one obese person in a thousand has a glandular problem, and frequently this malfunction is a consequence of obesity rather than its cause.

Although fashion models are getting thinner, studies show that most people are actually getting fatter. The National Center for Health Statistics reports that American women today weigh an average of almost thirteen pounds more than their counterparts did fifteen years ago: men, almost nine pounds more than the male average in 1960. And, according to the American Medical Association, at least 10 percent of all adult Americans are obese.

During the stages in life when heart attacks strike, people have a tendency to gain weight. Women are particularly prone to gain weight after menopause. Men usually add fat from age twenty-five to forty. As people get older, their overall metabolism slows down and caloric needs are reduced. So, to maintain at sixty the weight you had when you were twenty years old, you have to eat 20 percent less. Most people don't, thus increasing both their weight and their risk of heart attack.

You May Be Fatter than You Think

Interestingly, you may be overweight and not know it. In a 1979 study, over one million people across the country were surveyed by the Community Hypertension Evaluation Clinic: Men, especially young men, tended to underestimate their weight. Self-estimate of overweight was 19 percent in men under forty-five years old, compared with actual overweight of 35 percent; in men over forty-five, the self-estimate of overweight was 30 percent, compared with the actual overweight figure of 46 percent. These young men are precisely those most prone to heart attacks.

Test Yourself

How can you tell if you are too fat? Before you weigh yourself, try these simple tests:

1. *The ruler test.* Lie on your back and place a ruler on the abdomen along the midline of the body. If it points upward at the midsection, you probably are carrying too much fat.
2. *The pinch test.* With your thumb and forefinger, grasp a "pinch" of skin at the stomach, upper arm, buttocks and calf. Normally that pinch should be between one-half inch and one inch. A fold much more than one inch indicates excess fat.
3. *The mirror test.* Check the location of your fat. Is your fat the so-called android (manlike) kind of obesity with most of the fatty tissue above the waist, or a gynoid (womanlike) variety, concentrated below the waist? If you have these typical patterns, you probably are overweight.

Weigh Yourself

Now weigh yourself. The best time is before breakfast, without clothes, and after you have emptied your bladder and bowels. It is important to weigh yourself at the same time of day and under the same circumstances.

You should weigh yourself only once a week. Daily weight changes, usually related to fluid and salt intake, can be discouraging and misleading. In fact, people generally fluctuate three to five pounds in the course of a single day.

If you have decided to diet, the next step is keeping a record.

KEEP A RECORD

You should keep a weekly record of your weight. It will help you see exactly how your diet is progressing. This record will contain some depressing plateaus. Despite strict dieting, you may find you are not losing any weight. To stay at the same weight for a few days, even weeks, can be very discouraging. But it is important to understand this plateau phenomenon is not an unusual medical occurrence, although exactly why it happens is not known. It is known that eventually, if you ride out these plateaus, you will continue to lose weight.

WHAT SHOULD YOU WEIGH?

Below is a general guide to the most desirable weights for people twenty-five years and over. Weights are given for people without clothing and shoes since that is how most people usually weigh themselves.

*Desirable Weight Ranges for Adults**

MEN		WOMEN	
Height (In.)†	Weight (Lbs.)‡	Height (In.)†	Weight (Lbs.)‡
64	122–144	60	100–118
66	130–154	62	106–124
68	137–165	64	112–132
70	145–173	66	119–139
72	152–182	68	126–146
74	160–190	70	133–155

* Courtesy U. S. Department of Agriculture Information Bulletin No. 364
† Without shoes
‡ Without clothes

How to Lose Weight

There are no shortcuts to weight loss. "No matter what your age, genetic makeup or glandular state, the undeniable direct cause of overweight is overeating!" states Elizabeth M. Whelan, Executive Director of the American Council on Science and Health.

For safe and successful dieting, you should plan to lose about one-half but no more than two pounds a week. If twenty-five pounds below your present weight is your goal, plan to spread this loss over a three-month period.

Forget the Fads

Everyone warns against fad diets: "They're dangerous!" "They're unhealthy!" But why?

To put it simply, fads don't take off fat. They may, however, take off pounds. Dr. M. U. Yang, a member of the Clinical Metabolism section at St. Luke's Hospital in New York City explains, "People care too much about how many pounds they've lost instead of *what* the pounds consist of—fat, water, or muscle. It's far more important for permanent weight control to lose fat—only. Many people who lose too much water and sodium actually start to feel dizzy while standing or after rising from a reclining position."

Exercise Helps

In any discussion of diet and health, consistent exercise cannot be ignored. The key word is consistent. Exercise can only cause weight loss if it is done on a daily basis. If you consult a calorie/workout chart, you will realize that regular exercise will result in weight loss. For example, if you take a two-mile walk every day, you could lose roughly twenty-five pounds in one year—provided you don't increase your caloric intake.

Dinner Can Be Disastrous

"Obesity begins at 5:00 P.M.," warns Dr. Warren R. Guild, professor at Harvard Medical School and cardiologist at Peter Bent Brigham Hospital.

Usually the dieter is very good at breakfast and lunch. Breakfast might be only a cup of coffee and toast. Lunch may be salad and iced tea. But dinner brings downfall! A person may be starved due to his low food intake throughout the day. He might feel he "deserves" a nice dinner, so he sits longer and he eats more. A big meal undoes the day's efforts. Afterwards he feels guilty, wakes up guilty the next morning, has a small breakfast, and the cycle continues. A more even distribution of calories throughout the day will prevent this feeling of deprivation at dinner.

DIETING TRICKS

The following dieting tricks may help you control your appetite:

1. Put down the fork after each mouthful. People tend to eat more if they eat faster.
2. Eat in the dining room (rather than while reading a book, reclining, or watching television).
3. Do not leave food out on the kitchen counter.
4. Go grocery shopping after a large meal when you are not hungry.
5. Exercise right before dinner. A workout immediately prior to dinner can diminish or even abolish the desire for food.
6. Snack (carrots are ideal) shortly before dinner. Like Mother always said, it *will* kill your appetite.
7. Use a salad plate rather than a regular-size dinner plate.
8. Eat three meals a day. Don't skip breakfast and lunch and "make up for it at dinner." This can place excessive demands on the heart.
9. Eat between meals! Eat less, more often.
10. Restrict sugar. Most Americans eat 100 pounds of sugar a year. Stop using sugar and you're bound to start losing pounds.

The Salt Story

"Here's a low-salt diet for your husband, and don't forget, no salt at the table," your doctor may have said.

Why do most physicians recommend a low-salt or salt-free diet after a heart attack? Extra salt in the body raises blood pressure. Salt causes water retention. This extra fluid load leads to higher pressure in the arteries.

Studies show that among populations whose salt intake is very low, high blood pressure is virtually nonexistent. Studies of rats that are genetically destined for high blood pressure show that they develop high blood pressure and die at an earlier age when placed on a high salt diet. These same rats have a normal life span without high blood pressure if their diets are low in salt.

Your Daily Salt Intake

Now you might ask: Isn't some salt healthy? You may be surprised to learn that table salt—sodium chloride—is not an essential dietary additive. Most foods contain enough natural salt to fulfill your body's daily requirements for sodium. Yet Americans eat from two to five times more salt than they need each day. The average salt intake is about fifteen grams, or half an ounce a day. Your physician may suggest limiting your salt intake to two to five grams a day. This means no salt shaker at the table, avoiding salty foods, and cooking without salt.

Facts about Hidden Salt

Salt is put in many foods before they ever reach the shopping cart. Therefore, reading labels is extremely important although it can be difficult and time consuming. You should be aware that:

- One level teaspoon of MSG is about 750 mg of sodium (salt).
- Sodium cyclamate and sodium saccharin are often used in low-calorie foodstuffs.
- Sodium compounds are used to help cereals cook quickly or to give a smooth texture to chocolate products.
- Brine (salt and water) is used in canning vegetables, in making corned beef, pickles, and sauerkraut.

Sodium Compounds to Know About

Salt is frequently used in foods as part of a compound. When listed on food labels, the word "salt" does not always appear. The words "soda" or "sodium" or the symbol "Na" indicate that the product contains salt. Some of these compounds can be used without restriction (these are usually present in small amounts), others should be avoided:

Avoid	Use Without Worry
Brine	Disodium phosphate
Baking powder	Sodium alginate
Baking soda	Sodium propionate
	Sodium benzoate
	Sodium sulfite

Seasoning Without Salt

Most people feel salt makes food taste better. The secret of tasty food without salt is substitution.

Most of these seasonings contain one or more sodium compounds and should be avoided:

SEASONINGS TO AVOID

Celery salt	Chili sauce	Soy sauce
Garlic salt	Commercial bouillon	Worcestershire sauce
Onion salt	Barbecue sauces	Olives, pickles, relishes
Catsup	Meat tenderizers	Cooking wine

These seasonings should be substituted for salt:

SEASONINGS TO USE

For Beef	For Chicken	For Lamb
Bay leaf	Cranberries	Curry
Mustard	Lemon juice	Mint
Green pepper	Mushrooms	Rosemary
Mushrooms	Paprika	Garlic
Nutmeg	Parsley	Mustard
Onion	Thyme	
Lemon juice		
Pepper		
Thyme		

For Pork	For Fish	For Veal
Applesauce	Dill	Apricots
Pineapple	Lemon juice	Rosemary
Onion	Paprika	Lemon juice
Sage	Parsley	Paprika
	Tomato	

Some High-Sodium Foods to Avoid

Food	Portions	Sodium content (milligrams)
Baking soda	1 teaspoon	1,360
Bouillon	1 cup	782
Buttermilk	1 cup	312
Canned soups	1 cup	
Chicken noodle		979
Split pea		922
Vegetable beef		1,025
Canned spaghetti	1 cup	955
Cheeses	1 ounce	
American		210
American (processed)		341
Camembert (domestic)		210
Cheese spread (processed)		488
Roquefort		210
Swiss		213
Chow mein (canned)	½ cup	290
Cold cuts	1 ounce	390
Cookies (homemade)	1	
Chocolate chip		70
Sugar		32
Crab (canned)	¼ cup	400
Crackers	1	
Saltines		33
Soda		72
Doughnuts	1	175
Dried beef	1 ounce	1,290
Frankfurters	1	550
French fries (salted)	½ cup	276
Ham	1 ounce	330
Mustard (regular, prepared)	1 tablespoon	188
Olives	1	165
Pickles (dill)	1 large	714
Pie (fruit)	1 slice	452
Pizza	1 slice	647
Pot pies	1	
Beef		1,024
Turkey		876

Food	Portions	Sodium content (milligrams)
Salad dressings	1 tablespoon	
French		205
Italian		314
Roquefort		164
Sardines (canned)	1 ounce	247
Sauerkraut	½ cup	560
Soy sauce	1 tablespoon	1,099
TV dinners: chicken, fish, ham, meat loaf, swiss steak	1	Over 1,000
Vegetable juice	½ cup	240

The Complete Cholesterol Story

Heart attack victims have to watch not only calories and salt but cholesterol and fat, too. The average healthy American male should have a cholesterol level of 220 mg. If a person's cholesterol is higher, the risk of heart attack increases.

Atherosclerosis is related to fatty substances in the blood. The two most important fatty substances in the blood are cholesterol and triglycerides. Cholesterol comes from two sources:

1. It is made by the body.
2. It is obtained from animal fat and other saturated fats we eat.

Triglycerides come only from the foods we eat:

1. starches (grains)
2. carbohydrates (sweets)
3. fatty substances

When cholesterol, triglycerides, and calcium combine in the wall of a blood vessel, they form plaque deposits.

Atherosclerotic deposits have been produced in almost every species of laboratory animal—dogs, cats, pigs, chickens, ducks, pigeons, guinea pigs, hamsters, and monkeys—by feeding them high-fat, high-cholesterol foods. Monkeys have had heart attacks—including sudden fatal ones—similar to those that occur in humans when fed high-fat, high-cholesterol foods. These animal studies seem to indicate that diet, even more than stress and other factors, might be a leading cause of heart attacks.

Your Daily Cholesterol

Cholesterol is a normal part of every cell in our bodies, but too much cholesterol is dangerous. We might have too much cholesterol because we eat too many high-cholesterol foods.

Cholesterol is found only in foods of *animal* origin. It is not present in fruits, vegetables, cereal grains, vegetable oils, or other foods coming from plants.

Saturated fat intake can also cause atherosclerotic deposits in blood vessels. Saturated fat is found in all meats, but expensive meat—the more marbleized, prime grade—is higher in saturated fats. So the American Heart Association recommends that people purchase only the leanest meat available, trim all visible fat, and limit beef, lamb, and pork to three servings a week. Large amounts of saturated fat are also found in butter, cream, whole milk, and cheese. So these products should also be avoided in favor of low-fat substitutes.

Triglycerides are another cause of plaque build-up. When sugar is absorbed into the body, some of it is converted into fat particles called triglycerides. Foods that contain triglycerides are starches, sugars, and alcohol. Therefore, these should be limited.

Understanding Lipoproteins

Cholesterol and triglycerides are not soluble; they do not dissolve in water. These fats combine with proteins to create soluble substances called lipoproteins. Lipoproteins dissolve in the blood in different proportions of cholesterol and triglycerides. Too many lipoproteins in the blood create a condition called *hyper-lipidemia*, which leads to heart attacks. Blood tests can tell if hyper-lipidemia is present. There are five different types of hyper-lipidemia with different cholesterol/triglyceride proportions; Type II and Type IV are the most common.

TYPE II: Type II describes people who have very high cholesterol in the blood. They may have inherited a gene that leads to overproduction of cholesterol. It is very important that these people follow a low-cholesterol eating plan. If this doesn't work, drugs can be given which will bind the cholesterol in the intestines, so it is not absorbed in the circulation, but is excreted.

Scientists are now able to separate out from the blood a lipoprotein called high-density lipoprotein (HDL). HDL may be able to remove cholesterol from vessels and tissues and carry it back to the liver, where the cholesterol can be broken down for excretion. If your cholesterol is elevated but your HDL is at a high level as well, you will probably have less risk of developing atherosclerosis. As levels of HDL/cholesterol rise in the bloodstream, levels of triglycerides fall.

TYPE IV: In Type IV people, the triglyceride level is very high (the cholesterol is usually normal or slightly elevated). Most of these people also have abnormal glucose tolerance tests indicating a tendency to diabetes. Again, these people may be born with a gene that increases the triglyceride level. Diet is important. These people must cut down on carbohydrates (bread, pastries, pasta), sugar, and alcohol. A Type IV person can be given drugs, but sweets and liquor must still be avoided.

As mentioned earlier, excess intake of cholesterol raises the level of cholesterol in the blood. Therefore, the following foods containing high amounts of cholesterol and saturated fats should be avoided:

SOME HIGH-CHOLESTEROL, HIGH-FAT FOODS TO AVOID

Avocado	Cream	Milk, whole
Bacon	Light	Olives
Beef	Sour	
Brisket	Custard	Organ meats
Rib roast	Egg, yolk only	Liver
T-bone steak	Frozen or packaged dinners	Kidney
Butter	Ice cream	Peanut butter
Coconut	Lobster	Pork chops
		Potato chips

Four Rules of Low-Cholesterol Cooking

RULE #1: Use a roasting rack or ribbed-bottom skillet.

RULE #2: Trim all visible fat.

RULE #3: Use polyunsaturated oils (margarine, corn oil, and other vegetable oils) whenever possible.

RULE #4: Eat beef, lamb, pork, and ham only three times a week. Use fish and poultry (without skin) as often as possible.

Savory Substitutes

The secret of successful dieting is substitution. Some substitutes are so close in taste to the original product, it is often impossible to tell the difference. A famous cookbook writer and cholesterol watcher once served a delicious chocolate cake. "Chocolate is my only cholesterol vice," commented one guest. "I see you're the same way." He was amazed to learn that, in fact, the cake was both low in cholesterol and unbelievably delicious!

To give up fat without frustration, substitute:

- *polyunsaturated oils* for saturated oils
- *special margarine* for butter or hydrogenated shortenings
- *evaporated skim milk* for light cream
- *skim milk* for whole milk
- *cocoa* for unsweetened chocolate (substitute 2½ tablespoons cocoa plus 1½ teaspoons safflower oil for one square unsweetened chocolate)
- *partially skim-milk cheese* for whole-milk cheese (partially skim-milk cheese is not fat-free and should be used sparingly, however)

Oils to Use

Polyunsaturated fats tend to lower the level of cholesterol in the blood by helping the body to eliminate excess, newly formed cholesterol. Generally, polyunsaturated fats are liquid at room temperature. The following oils are high in polyunsaturated fats and should be used:

- corn oil
- cottonseed oil
- safflower oil
- sesame seed oil
- soybean oil
- sunflower oil
- walnut oil

(Walnut oil is the most highly polyunsaturated of all the oils but is not readily available. The next most highly polyunsaturated oil is safflower oil, which is readily available and should be used often.)

Oils to Avoid

The following oils should be avoided:

Coconut oil

Of all the oils, coconut oil is the highest in fatty acids. Because of its good keeping quality, it is frequently used in commercially baked goods, candy, imitation whipped toppings, and fried or roasted products such as potato chips and nuts. These products should be avoided.

Cocoa butter

Cocoa butter, the main ingredient in chocolate should be avoided. Cocoa powder, which is chocolate with much of the cocoa butter removed, should be used in place of chocolate.

Solid and hydrogenated oil

Hydrogenated oils—vegetable oils that have been hardened by a process called *hydrogenation*—should be avoided because this process converts some polyunsaturated fats to monounsaturated and saturated fats. The following products contain large amounts of saturated fats: hydrogenated vegetable shortenings, lard, imitation whipped creams, and palm oil (often used in commercially prepared baked goods).

Eating Out: The Better Way

Most people eat out at least once a week. You can enjoy your restaurant meals without worry by knowing what to select and how to order it.

The all-American dinner is:

Shrimp cocktail
Steak, rare

Baked potato with sour cream and bacon bits
Salad with blue cheese dressing
Coconut cream pie

Your mouth is watering—but you know it's poison. One leading cardiologist suggests, "Pretend the foods actually contain arsenic; it's easier to resist that way." You can enjoy basically the same meal with a few changes but a big difference in total calories, cholesterol, saturated fats, and triglycerides. You should order:

Grapefruit
Steak, well trimmed and broiled without fat
Baked potato with margarine
Salad with pepper and lemon juice
Lemon sherbet

Breakfast out is usually no problem: Order cereal with skim milk, bran or corn muffins with margarine; avoid french toast, waffles, and eggs. For lunch, order fruit salad or chef salad; avoid cheeseburgers, hot dogs, and tuna fish. Dinner can present problems. Here's a dining-out guide for enjoyable evening meals.

Your Menu Guide

APPETIZERS

Order: tomato juice, raw vegetables, shrimp cocktail (occasionally), fruit cup
Avoid: avocado, caviar, anchovies, salmon, cream cheese, all cheeses, creamed soups

ENTRÉES

Order: fish, chicken or veal—ask that they be broiled without fat
Avoid: beef and all meats made with cream or egg-based sauces such as Newburg, or Béarnaise

VEGETABLES

Order: any fresh, frozen, or canned plain vegetables
Avoid: any vegetables cooked in cream sauce, butter sauce, or sautéed

SALAD

Order: any green or fruit salad. Use lemon juice or vinegar dressing

Avoid: prepared salad dressings

BREAD

Order: plain sliced bread or hard rolls with margarine

Avoid: biscuits, popovers, and muffins because they were probably made with saturated fat

BEVERAGE

Order: skim milk, coffee, tea, fruit juice

Avoid: soda, whole milk, and cream

DESSERT

Order: jello, fruit, sherbet, ices, angel food cake

Avoid: creamed custards, whipped cream, pies, and cakes

It Does Make a Difference

"I'm doomed—it just doesn't matter—my heart will get me eventually." This kind of thinking is not only pessimistic, but more importantly, it is incorrect. Your weight can make a tremendous difference in your chances of having another heart attack.

These sobering statistics should be remembered:

- A fifty-year-old man who is fifty pounds overweight has only half the life expectancy of a man the same age with normal weight.
- A man has a seven times greater chance of developing coronary heart disease if his cholesterol is above 259 rather than below 200.

You Can Do It

Going on a diet for a few weeks or months can be trying. Life-long dieting—the kind required for heart patients—is extremely difficult. Statistics confirm that only 20 percent of the people who are overweight will be able to lose those extra pounds.

Proper weight means looking better, feeling better, and being healthier. It is important for everyone. For the person who has had a heart attack, it is vital.

12. Tennis, Anyone?

YEARS AGO, a heart attack meant an armchair existence.

"My father had a heart attack when he was thirty-eight," one middle-aged man recalled. "Until he died eight years later, he lived the life of an invalid. Once—just once—in those eight years I remember seeing him toss a football. The rest of the time he sat quietly, read, listened to music, and (as I came to realize much later) put his affairs in order."

Today, doctors and patients alike do not believe in quietly giving up. They've started to fight, and one of their most effective weapons is exercise.

What People Say

People rave about it. "We're impossible—worse than missionaries," joked a fifty-year-old man who suffered two heart attacks and now runs three miles a day, rain or shine. When asked what drives them to pursue with a passion what many regard as little more than socially accepted masochism, people say such things as: "I feel like a new person"; "I sleep better"; "I eat less"; "My complexion is better"; "I'm more relaxed"; "I don't get so upset anymore"; "I feel sexier."

Dr. George Sheehan, cardiologist and renowned runner, agrees. "If I were trying to get people to be more productive on the job, I'd give them all sweat suits and then send them running at lunchtime. For me, my stream of consciousness becomes a torrent when I run. New ideas and thoughts come pouring in. We all went wrong in the eighth grade, when we put our bodies behind desks and concentrated on what the mind can do. Luckily some genius discovered recess."

It sounds great, but does it really work? Can exercise really help the heart or prevent heart attacks? Does it improve the chances of surviving a heart attack and prolong life?

Unfortunately, definitive answers are just not known, but current evidence suggests that exercise—if practiced sensibly according to a personally tailored exercise "prescription"—can help the heart. The American Heart Association advises that exercise is "prudent."

Sneakers and Medical Studies

For years, studies have shown that regular exercise can reduce the risk of heart disease while inactivity may actually increase this risk. In 1958, Paul Dudley White and William C. Pomeroy did an interesting study of 335 former athletes. It was found that none of those who continued to exercise after retiring suffered heart attacks. However, of the retired athletes who did not exercise, about a third died of heart attacks.

In an English study, bus conductors who climbed up and down double-decker buses had less heart disease than the inactive drivers of the same buses.

In the United States, a similar study of 120,000 railroad workers found that inactive office workers suffered twice as many heart attacks as more active yard workers.

The longest running (twenty-two years) and most recently completed (late 1979) report, called the "Longshoreman's Study," documented the benefit of exercise on the heart. Thirty-six hundred longshoremen between the ages of thirty-five and fifty-four, were studied in San Francisco. Those who worked at strenuous jobs had the lowest risk of a fatal heart attack, while those who worked at less active jobs ran three times the risk of a fatal heart attack. The combination of a sedentary lifestyle, heavy smoking, and high blood pressure increased by as much as twenty times the risk of a fatal heart attack!

Naturally, exercise is not a cure-all. Dr. Remington, dean of the University of Michigan School of Public Health, has said,

"Someone who thinks he's protecting his heart by running around the track several times a week but continues to eat a high-fat diet or smoke two packs a day is just kidding himself. Many factors combine to cause heart disease. Physical activity probably does have a protective effect, but it has to be integrated into a healthful lifestyle."

A fascinating study of lumberjacks in East Finland dramatized this. These men are extremely active, expending many thousands of calories a week, but their diet is very high in saturated fats and cholesterol. The result: Their death rate from heart disease is the highest of any population yet studied.

Excuses, Excuses

"Next week, I'll do it."

"I just don't have the time."

"I don't believe in artificially waving your arms around."

"That's for young kids. Not me."

"It's just a fad. It'll fade like the hula-hoop!"

"I'm too lazy."

"I'm taking a few days off from that damn bike."

We all know the excuses. A few people really believe exercise is bad for you; somehow, they imagine, exercise enlarges the heart. While athletes *do* have large hearts, this cannot happen to the average person even if he exercises three to four times a week. "Athlete's heart" only occurs in those who do vigorous exercise every single day, and for these athletes, a large heart is neither abnormal nor dangerous.

Another erroneous idea is that everyday living provides sufficient exercise and it isn't necessary to do anything more. This is just not so.

"Oh, I'm much too old for that!" many men and women over fifty assume. This is a serious misconception. Many experts now believe that older people have a special need for exercise. A study by two Israeli psychologists developed the theory that while young children love to move, older people sometimes feel that "proper" behavior means they should not "move around like children." They are expected to be "dignified," and eventually, they may be reluctant to move at all. This Israeli study further suggested that a distortion of body image may result. Physically inactive people over fifty, they found, perceive their bodies to be heavier and broader than they really are. Therefore, many elderly people come to incorrectly assume exercise is too strenuous for them.

Time is the most common excuse. Interestingly, the Perrier Study—the first survey of fitness in America since 1961—showed that when "low actives" and "high actives" compared their available free time, it was almost exactly the same—about twenty-five hours a week.

The outstanding reason "non-actives" in the Perrier Study gave for beginning a program was a doctor's advice, although many enjoyed it much more than they had imagined. As one man put it, "I used to growl about walking; I'd take the car down to the corner for a newspaper. After walking became a habit, I've gotten to like it. Even on the golf course, I don't use a cart."

A reminder:

If you stop exercising for a time, the benefits are not maintained. In restarting to exercise, begin again slowly and build up gradually. Do not start at the level where you left off months earlier.

When to Begin

Start early! is today's dictum. Dr. Wenger, chairman of the rehabilitation committee of the American Heart Association has said, "Supervised low-level physical activity for the patient with uncomplicated myocardial infarction may begin as early as the first days in the coronary care unit."

Dr. Rubenstein usually tells his patients, "In the first few days home, begin to do normal life activities—dressing, showering, shaving, helping around the house. After a day or two, start walking. Walk to the end of your street and back. By the second week, go around the block, then try a few blocks. After two months, ask your doctor about a stress test. Gradually set up a more active schedule. It all comes with time. Don't overdo, and know when to stop. Angina, shortness of breath or fatigue, again, are all red lights."

Early exercise helps relieve anxiety and depression so common after a heart attack. It may prevent dizziness and rapid heartbeat which often occur when people on prolonged bed rest first try to stand and walk. It decreases the risk of blood clots. And importantly, it shows the person his heart is healing and that he will be able to resume a normal or near normal lifestyle. It has immense psychological value.

Before exercising it is essential to have a complete checkup, even if you have no complaints. A checkup includes a physical examination, lab work, and usually a stress test. Data has shown that most people can safely take a stress test two to three months after an uncomplicated heart attack. The results of this complete examination provide a guide for continuing activity levels.

Your Stress Test

"Ready for your test, Mrs. Goldstein?" Dr. Rubenstein asked. Two months before, Mrs. Goldstein had suffered an uncomplicated myocardial infarction at age fifty-nine and now was eager to return to playing golf in Florida. Her stress test was typical of those given after a heart attack. Her appointment was for 10:00 A.M. and the doctor had told her it would last about an hour.

"The nurse will show you where you can change into your shorts, sneakers, shirt, and cotton bra." Synthetics can cause static electrical interference, the doctor told her. Mrs. Goldstein had not eaten breakfast since she had been told "no food or heavy liquids for at least five hours before the test."

In the examining room, Mrs. Goldstein saw a machine the size of a doctor's upright scale. But instead of the stand to weigh yourself, there was a treadmill with a four-foot-long conveyor belt on which to walk. The treadmill can be tilted to simulate a hill and adjusted for speed.

Mrs. Goldstein was shown how to walk on the moving belt, balancing by lightly holding onto the stabilizing bar in front. "The machine will gradually go faster, but be sure to tell us at the slightest sign of any discomfort, shortness of breath, weakness, or any unusual feelings," he doctor explained.

The nurse prepared the skin for the electrodes by rubbing gently with acetone or alcohol. It caused a slight burning sensation. "This is the only discomfort in the test," the nurse said. "And be glad you're not a man. To get the electrodes to stick on them, we sometimes have to shave spots on their chests!" The nurse then placed small, foam rubber, sticky electrodes on her body—some on the chest, the middle of the back, and one on each arm and leg.

The doctor watched the cardiogram closely as Mrs. Goldstein walked. He checked her blood pressure frequently and he asked if there were any pain in the chest or shortness of breath. Mrs. Goldstein was trying hard as she walked briskly. Dr. Rubenstein was testing the level at which her heart could work without distress. The test shows if the heart is getting adequate oxygen even under stress. An adequate oxygen supply means that blood is flowing through the arteries or collateral arteries as it should.

Mrs. Goldstein completed the test, tired but pleased.

"But why did I really need all of this?" she asked.

"Even though a coronary artery is severely narrowed, the heart may still get enough oxygen at rest, and the resting cardiogram may be acceptable," Dr. Rubenstein said. "But with stress from the treadmill the demands on the heart increase and possible problems will become apparent. But you're fine. So enjoy your golf and let your husband win a few games!"

How to Begin

There are four things to consider when starting an exercise program: your age, your weight, your prior inactivity level, and your health status. Let's consider each.

- *Your age:* with advancing age, you have to be more careful about the level at which you start exercising.
- *Your weight:* excessive weight requires greater effort in exercise.

A warning:

Exercise tests themselves have rarely caused heart attacks. The rare heart attacks that have occurred probably would have happened if exercise had been done without a test. It is important to mention that stress tests can occasionally give misleading results. The test may be considered positive if the person develops EKG abnormalities. False positive tests, more common in younger women, can have crippling psychological effects. A false negative may cause people to overestimate their exercise capacity. So all tests should be done under the close supervision of an experienced cardiologist and in collaboration with other diagnostic studies and clinical impressions.

- *Your prior inactivity:* the longer you have been inactive, the less able you are to initially perform certain levels of exercise.
- *Your health status:* this affects the level of exercise you can safely do.

Everyone given the green light to exercise should start slowly and over a period of weeks increase the strenuousness of the exercise.

Each exercise period—ideally lasting around twenty minutes —should begin with a five- to ten-minute warm-up and end with a five- to ten-minute cool-down. Even though you are tempted, don't collapse into a chair or stand immobile at the end of your exercise program.

To help the heart, exercise levels must fall between 70 and 85 percent of your maximal heart or pulse rate. Take your pulse after each exercise to be sure you are performing the proper amount of exercise.

To get an idea of average maximal heart rate, you can calculate it roughly by subtracting your age in years from the number 220.

Thus, if you are forty-five years old, your maximal heart rate would theoretically be 175, and the pulse rate to aim for—your target zone—would be between 122 and 148 beats per minute. To determine whether you've reached your target zone, take your pulse immediately upon stopping exercise by counting the beats for ten seconds and multiplying by six.

For those who have had a heart attack, however, normal heart rate means little. It is imperative that you only exercise to the point recommended by your doctor.

Your Exercise Timetable

A good time to exercise is in the morning before breakfast; another good time is before dinner. However, in both cases, rest for ten to fifteen minutes before sitting down to eat. Doctors say the time of day is generally unimportant, but you should never exercise directly after eating, after missing several meals, or when exhausted or ill.

Selecting a Sport

"The exercise that benefits you most is the exercise you do," advises Charles Kuntzelman in *The Complete Book of Running*.

Doctors say, "Pick something you like." Looking back to happy childhood memories sometimes gives people ideas.

After a heart attack, some forms of exercise should, however, be avoided. There are two types of sports: rhythmic and static (isometric). Rhythmic sports require long, steady, sustained movements that are very beneficial to the heart. Static sports require short, rapid, forceful movements, that can be dangerous for anyone with a heart problem. They increase heart rate, blood pressure, and can even cause a heart attack. Winston Churchill suffered a mild heart attack after straining to open a White House window (a static movement) during a visit to Washington.

You don't have to pick a popular sport. Indeed, it might surprise you to learn that a recent Harris Poll showed that the most popular sport in America today is not tennis or running. It's walking! (Swimming and calisthenics are next.) And this is precisely what most doctors recommend right after a heart attack.

Contrary to popular belief, Dr. Lenore Zohman, an exercise cardiologist at Montefiore Hospital points out, "There is no best exercise for everyone. If you have an aversion to organized sports or strenuous activity, brisk walking for twenty or thirty minutes or climbing up stairs at a comfortable pace during a day can help achieve physical fitness."

Exercise does not have to be expensive, time-consuming or organized. For example, jumping rope takes little time, no partner, and costs nothing. According to Sidney Filson, author and rope-jumping instructor, there is nothing you can spend less time on that gives you more results. For example, tests done over a six-week period compared cardiovascular gain with rope jumping over other sports and found that fifteen minutes of rope jumping is equivalent to three sets of tennis singles, thirty-seven holes of golf, one hour of snow or water skiing, and one and a half hours of roller skating. Rope jumping must never be done without first discussing it with your cardiologist.

The following guide will help you select other beneficial sports.

Select: Sports requiring a good deal of running or repeated continuous movement:

jogging	stationary cycling
running	tennis
cycling	basketball
swimming	skating (indoors)
dancing	hiking
brisk walking	golf
table tennis	badminton

Avoid: Sports requiring long pauses or spurts of activity:

weight-lifting	baseball
water skiing	football
snow skiing	soccer
bowling	

Even some hobbies can provide excellent exercise. Carpentry, for example, uses gross movements and gives a feeling of creativity in addition.

Outdoor photography and bird-watching can involve extensive walking. Gardening is great; you bend, you dig, and again exercise is involved. (Just avoid extremely hot weather and hot sun.)

Remember, the key to fitness training is heart rate, not a pre-conceived notion of what constitutes exercise. A dull game of tennis doubles or a slow eighteen holes of golf might be fun, but it probably will not have an effect on heart rate.

Working Up a Sweat

For exercise to have an effect on the heart, doctors advise that a person should "work up a sweat for twenty minutes at least three times a week." Exercise should be divided into two- to four-minute blocks of activity with one to two minutes of recovery in between.

It is important to exercise regularly, not in fits and starts. The weekend tennis player or weekend jogger cannot optimally achieve a training effect. Doctors usually recommend exercising every other day, using Sunday as a catch-up day if a day is missed.

The older the person, the less rigorous the activity required to produce a beneficial effect on the heart.

Does It Work?

The examples are indisputable:

1. At Barnes Hospital in St. Louis, Howard Palliz, a patient in his early fifties, could shuffle through only seven short laps around the track after his heart attack. Within six weeks, he was doing thirty-four.
2. At Greenwich Hospital in Connecticut, one patient could hardly walk two blocks when he joined the program. Eventually he ran a mile nonstop in eleven minutes.
3. In George Washington Hospital in Washington, a group of chronically ill heart patients—ages sixty-five to eighty-five—performed vigorous calisthenics for some U.S. senators. While heart disease had made them almost completely immobile, after exercising only six months they were once again participating in life, rather than sitting on the sidelines.

Nothing can make heart attack damage disappear, but exercise can improve heart function. It can dramatically change the way a person feels, looks and acts.

A Healed Heart

According to Dr. Lenore Zohman, the main cardiovascular benefit of exercise is that it improves the efficiency of the heart. The heart can pump more blood with less effort, and rest longer between beats. So the heart does not have to work as hard.

A person who exercises regularly has a lower heart rate at a given level of exercise. He can exercise vigorously for a longer time without feeling tired and can respond to sudden physical and emotional demands without his heart racing or his blood pressure rising precipitously.

Exercise also lowers blood pressure (pressure rises during exercise but is lower at rest). The flow of blood to the lungs and muscles is increased. Auxiliary circulation within the heart may increase, and possibly some of the atherosclerotic plaque may disappear due to the effect of exercise on lipoproteins.

These changes go by various names: cardiovascular enhancement, increased aerobic capacity, the training effect. Very simply, people feel like they have more wind, more stamina, more endurance.

More Lipoproteins: Less Cholesterol

New studies have also shown that regular exercise increases the level of high-density lipoproteins in the blood. People with high levels of lipoproteins, or HDL, are far less prone to heart disease than the average person.

"Physical activity seems to be the best way to increase HDL levels," explains Dr. William L. Haskell of Stanford University. His studies of 4,600 men and women showed that exercise itself raised HDL levels. In fact, exercise increased this type of lipoprotein that is naturally higher in women than in men and is believed to be one reason women are relatively immune to heart attacks before menopause.

Exercise also affects cholesterol. HDL seems to remove cholesterol from arteries and encourage its excretion. An active person who watches his saturated fat intake can more easily maintain normal serum cholesterol levels than a sedentary person.

As Dr. John L. Boyer, medical director of the California State University Coronary Rehabilitation Center has stated, "Once someone begins to improve on one of his coronary risk factors, he'll work on others. This is one of the most important and far-reaching reasons you should encourage patients to exercise."

More Muscle . . . Less Fat

Exercise helps people lose unwanted pounds and keep them off. Dr. Leonard Epstein of Western Psychiatric Institute in Pittsburgh has reported that people who both exercise and diet lose more weight and are more likely to continue to lose than those who simply diet.

A recent study showed that a 170-pound man who runs a mile and a half in eight minutes burns 175 calories. Someone who does this regularly—without an increase in caloric intake—can lose ten pounds in a year.

The benefit is not so much a change in body weight as it is a change in body fat. The person who exercises is likely to be slimmer even if there is no weight loss, because fat is replaced by muscle. Muscle is denser than fat; therefore, muscle of a given weight takes up less room than fat of the same weight.

A Look at an Exercise Center

To see just what an exercise program was like, I visited the 92nd Street YM & YWHA in New York City, which has a well-known Coronary Detection and Intervention Center.

If I hadn't been told that the participants had once been seriously ill, I would never have believed it. Two or three were only in their thirties—slim, trim, and athletic looking. There were two attractive women in their late forties; the rest were an even sprinkling of men in their forties, fifties, and sixties.

I spoke with Chuck Bronze, a soft-spoken man in his early forties, who developed and directs the program. He told me classes meet for an hour, three times a week. There is no organized sport. Each person follows an individually planned exercise program based on a stress test given by a cardiologist at the beginning of the program. Five months later, another stress test is given to see if improvement has been made. To find out who was there and why, I spoke with some of the participants. Here's what they said:

Wade Morrison
Age: 55
Occupation: Liquor executive
Medical History: One heart attack while playing indoor tennis
Appearance: 6′1″, muscular, ruggedly handsome

"I was an athlete before, always kept myself in shape by skiing, baseball, and swimming.

"No, I never dreamed it would happen to me, but when it did, I knew I'd get back into shape. I had my attack in July on the tennis court and was skiing six months later.

"My endurance has definitely improved. Last winter when I went skiing, I'd get a few yards and stop and puff. Now I have no problem with my wind."

Dan Jopheson
Age: 35
Occupation: Advertising executive
Medical History: A bypass operation at age 34
Appearance: Bearded, slight, youthful, and intense

"I love to exercise, but I'm not self-disciplined. I was very motivated at the beginning but it's hard to keep it up. It's an excellent program as long as you stay with it."

Jack Wilson
Age: 50
Occupation: Attorney
Medical History: One heart attack at age 48
Appearance: Medium build, receding hairline, serious

"I come after work, by subway, three days a week, five-fifteen to six o'clock. I'd rather go home but it's something I know I must do.

"What do I do? I do sixty-five seconds of jumping jacks, eighty seconds up and down seventeen steps, seventy-five seconds of rope jump. I jog twenty-four laps on the track, do thirty sit-ups, and run five laps at moderate speed. I do twenty-four medicine-ball tosses in a circle, and then I run four laps fast."

Jane Windamere
Age: 55
Occupation: Librarian
Medical History: One possible heart attack and a history of rapid pulse and heart murmurs since childhood
Appearance: Tweedy, soft-spoken, slightly nervous

"I'm a tense person—more so than average, I think. And I've always tired easily. Exercising definitely gives me more energy; I sleep better; I eat more and I think I feel better all around. My only complaint is I've gained weight. All this work makes me hungry, and I've got no resistance at all: I eat!"

Psychological Benefits of Exercise

The psychological benefits of exercise are enormous. People feel better, they look better and they enjoy life more. Furthermore, in practically all cases, their sex lives improve.

Dr. Terence Kavanaugh, director of one of the most highly regarded cardiac rehabilitation programs has stated, "One third of a sample of our patients had neurotic type personalities and developed excessive depression after a heart attack. In most cases, patients became less depressed as they exercised more."

Unquestionably, people who exercise will gain feelings of self-control. They become less afraid to do things—more willing to participate fully in life. Exercise has a social side, too; there is a feeling of camaraderie. Discussions about shoes, outfits, and competitions are easy. Illness tends to intensify loneliness and isolation, so this social interchange is extremely beneficial.

People who exercise soon make small changes in their daily life. They use stairs instead of elevators, walk instead of ride, and walk faster rather than slower. These daily changes also benefit the heart.

Know When to Stop

Even with a clean bill of health and proper precautions, some symptoms may occur during exercise, especially at the outset.

"If I feel chest pain or winded while exercising, should I stop or continue, hoping it will disappear?" many people ask. Doctors say it is imperative to *stop immediately*. Any feelings of pressure or burning in the center of the chest or behind the breastbone, or strange indigestion pains during or immediately after exercise, lasting from a few minutes to several minutes, are a sign to stop immediately and call your doctor.

All exercise, at least initially, must be followed by taking your own heart rate. If a particular exercise leads to rapid heart rate increase or rhythm disturbance, it should be discontinued at once.

Symptoms which occur several hours after exercise are usually less significant than those which occur during or immediately after exercise.

Things to Avoid

"Exercise is like a drug," Dr. Herman K. Hellerstein, professor of medicine at Case Western Reserve University in Cleveland, warns. "It has a dosage, frequency, complications, indications, and contraindications. Like any drug, exercise can be abused as well as used in health-saving ways."

New exercise converts often do themselves more harm than good. To avoid undue stress on the heart, the following DON'TS must be observed.

DON'T:

· Exercise—even walking—in very cold, very hot, or very humid weather.
· Swim in very cold water. Enter the water gradually.
· Exercise when tired or stressed or ill.
· Exercise immediately after eating.
· Exercise at high altitudes.

"Four out of seven guys in the CCU with me were taken off tennis courts," one heart attack victim told us. Sudden exercise spurts can be dangerous; all exercise after a heart attack must be done under a doctor's guidance.

For Further Information

Before embarking on a serious exercise program, you might benefit from information provided in the following books.

Dr. Lenore Zohman's pamphlet, *Beyond Diet . . . Exercise Your Way to Fitness and Heart Health* is an excellent basic primer about all types of exercise and how to go about an exercise program. Single copies can be obtained free by writing Mazola Nutrition Information Service, Dept. ZD-NYT, Box 307, Coventry, CT 06238.

Dr. Kenneth H. Cooper's book *Aerobics,* published in paperback by Bantam in 1968, has been a bestseller ever since. Aerobic exercises—running, walking, jogging, cycling, swimming, and rope jumping—all strengthen the heart. Besides this basic text, Dr. Cooper has also written *Aerobics for Women* and *The New Aerobics,* both excellent reading.

I3. Everything You Should Know about Your Heart Medicines

"I NEVER TOOK a pill before my heart attack and I don't take any now either," a thirty-eight-year-old heart attack victim told us. After a heart attack, some people don't need any pills. Doctors say, however, very few escape pill-free. Most people are given some prescriptions before leaving the hospital.

Pills are powerful; they can do immense good, but they can also be harmful. It is essential that people know about the pills they are taking. Regardless of the type of drug, some basic pill-taking rules should be followed.

Pill-taking Rules

RULE #1: Take your pills *regularly*. Certain drugs for the heart can be dangerous if their use is interrupted.

RULE #2: Don't stop taking a pill even if you feel well or run out of pills. Renew at once. Don't wait for your next visit to the doctor.

RULE #3: Follow your doctor's orders precisely. Certain heart drugs must be taken in the exact dosage and frequency prescribed. Varying dosages can be extremely dangerous.

RULE #4: If you experience a side effect, don't just stop the medicine. Call your doctor immediately for advice.

RULE #5: Don't take any drug at all—even the most apparently harmless that has nothing to do with the heart—without consulting your doctor. Sometimes drugs taken together can have serious side effects that neither has alone. For example, if you are taking a drug to reduce the risk of a blood clot, and take aspirin for some minor pain, the result may be severe bleeding.

Pill-taking Tricks

If you've recently been sick, undoubtedly you're not as organized as usual. How do you remember everything when it all seems so new, so scary, and so confusing. Again, we've asked the men and women who've had the problem. Here's what they said:

"I put my pills in all different places around the house—near the TV, near the phone, by my bed, on the kitchen table. Right beneath the bottle I wrote directions for how much and when. Then if I don't feel well, my husband can just read the directions. It saves steps, uncertainty, and arguments too."

"I keep an alarm clock in the office. At nine, twelve, and four —pill times—it goes off. I usually don't forget, but this way I never forget."

"One day, I went around putting my pills in all my coat pockets, and I put some in the glove compartment of the car. Also, I bought a special key case where a few pills can fit, so I don't have to constantly remember to take them along."

"Believe it or not, my wife made a notebook with lined charts and I make an 'x' in the column each time I take a pill. I leave the notebook on the kitchen table."

"I keep one day's supply in a little brown bottle. Sometimes if I'm busy I can't remember if I've taken a pill or not, and this system keeps track for me. My doctor recommended it and I really find it helps."

The Most Common Heart Drugs

Digitalis, nitroglycerin, Inderal, and Coumadin are familiar names to most people after a heart attack. Here's how and why they may be prescribed.

Digitalis

Digitalis, one of the oldest drugs in the doctor's bag, was first discovered by an Englishwoman who mixed herbs together to treat dropsy. Digoxin is the form most commonly prescribed because of its rapid and reliable action.

How It Looks: Digoxin comes in yellow tablets (.125 milligrams), white tablets (.25 mg) and green tablets (.5 mg).

What It Does: Digitalis works in two ways. First, it enables the heart to pump more blood with each beat. Second, it regulates and regularizes the heart's contraction rate. This usually brings a radical improvement in the person's condition.

Who Should Take It: Not everyone after a heart attack needs digitalis. It is used specifically for people with congestive heart failure because it helps eliminate excess fluid in the body due to poor pumping efficiency. It is also prescribed for people with rapid heartbeat because it regulates and slows the abnormal rhythms.

How Much Should You Take? It depends on your age and weight. A smaller dose is usually used for older, thinner, and smaller people.

However digitalis must be taken only under close medical supervision since many other factors can affect the drug's efficiency. For example, if the person is also taking diuretics, which cause a larger excretion of sodium and potassium in the urine, the risk of side effects increases. Therefore, the doctor may recommend eating a banana each day (they are rich in potassium) or taking a potassium supplement.

The dosage of digitalis may be high during the first day or two of its use. This is called the "digitalizing dose." Once "digitalized" properly, a smaller maintenance dose is taken once or twice a day.

Possible Side Effects: If you absorb or take too much digitalis, digitalis overdose can occur. The early warning signs of overdose include appetite loss, nausea, vomiting, sometimes diarrhea, and weakness.

If any of these side effects occur, your doctor should be notified promptly. This is very important because if the drug is continued, irregularities of the heartbeat may result.

Even rarer symptoms of overdose are allergic skin rashes,

breast enlargement (even in men, in one or both breasts), spots before the eyes, or a flickering sensation.

Your physician can monitor the dose of digitalis by taking blood samples for a test that shows the level of the drug present in your system. Blood tests alone are not always definitive. With a review of symptoms and a physical examination, however, proper dosage can be determined (sometimes blood tests are not necessary).

Be aware:

1. Digitalis should not be taken on an empty stomach.
2. No antacids should be taken within six hours after digitalis.
3. Never discontinue digitalis or change the dose without the advice of a physician.
4. When refilling the prescription, never repeat the initial digitalization dose; simply continue the maintenance dose.

Nitroglycerin

Nitroglycerin, usually prescribed to overcome attacks of angina, works remarkably fast, often producing almost instantaneous relief. It is also used to prevent angina attacks.

"It's like a truck going up hill," explained Dr. Marshall Franklin, a Connecticut cardiologist and author of *The Doctor's Heart Book*. "A truck with a partly blocked gas line can just make it on level ground. Well, nitroglycerin smooths out the hill (decreases the work load) . . . and the patient reaches the crest."

How It Looks: Nitro, as people often call it, comes most commonly in small white tablets.

There is also a nitroglycerin paste. It is applied on strips of paper to the skin and is particularly helpful when angina wakes you in the middle of the night. When applied before going to sleep, nitro paste may prevent such attacks. It provides longer lasting relief than the pills (up to several hours).

What It Does: A unique pill, nitroglycerin, per se, does little good if swallowed. It should be placed under the tongue when chest pain occurs (or when it is anticipated). It is dissolved by saliva and rapidly absorbed.

Nitroglycerin relieves anginal pain remarkably fast. Doctors believe it works by expanding the venous blood vessels in the rest of the body. This decreases the amount of work done by the heart.

How Much Should You Take? Nitroglycerin is not habit forming; one should not hesitate to take it. Nitro should be taken as often as pain recurs or when entering situations that might provoke an angina attack. It is much better to take nitroglycerin than have the heart experience angina. Unrelieved angina can eventually damage the heart.

If the first nitroglycerin does not give relief, another should be taken in two to three minutes. If there is still pain, a third nitroglycerin should be taken after two or three minutes. However, doctors caution, three pills is enough. If pain continues, you should call your doctor immediately and go to the nearest emergency room. It may be a false alarm, but in case of emergency, a hospital can always provide the best possible care.

Possible Side Effects: A pounding headache for a short time may be caused by expansion of the blood vessels in the brain. There also may be a harmless flushing of the face or a light burning sensation under the tongue. These side effects become milder after the tablets have been taken for a while.

While annoying, these possible side effects are certainly worth bearing measured against the great relief given by nitroglycerin.

Anticoagulants

Anticoagulants interfere with the tendency of blood to clot. There are two kinds of anticoagulants. One is Heparin. The other is Coumadin. The choice depends on various medical circumstances.

How It Looks: Heparin is given by injection. If it is needed over the long-term, people are taught how to inject it much as diabetic

Be aware:
1. Always keep nitroglycerin in a dark, tightly closed bottle with a screw cap.
2. Get new nitroglycerin every three months. Nitroglycerin spoils, evaporates, and loses its potency. It should cause a slight burning sensation when placed under your tongue. If it doesn't, discard it and buy a fresh supply.
3. Nitroglycerin is absorbed by cotton and paper. Never put cotton in the pill bottle. Never put the label inside. As one doctor said, "We can't tell you how many patients we have seen who store nitroglycerin in plastic, snap-top containers filled with cotton with the paper label inside. After a week or two they might just as well chew the cotton as take the nitroglycerin."
4. Take nitroglycerin while sitting or lying down. Sometimes dizziness or faintness can occur if it is taken while standing.
5. You should take nitroglycerin for all cardiac pain, not just chest pain. It works for cardiac pain in the throat, jaws, gums, lower teeth, shoulders, between the shoulders and back, and down the arms.
6. Call your doctor if pain recurs many times during a day. Frequently recurring angina—especially if it has not occurred before—should be treated in a hospital.

patients are taught how to administer their own insulin. Heparin is given by injection either directly into the vein every four hours or just under the skin every eight to twelve hours. Coumadin is taken as a pill, just once a day.

How It Works: Heparin works by directly interfering with the chemical steps that make blood clot. Coumadin prevents the liver from producing prothrombin. It is prothrombin in the blood that helps blood clot.

Who Should Take It? Years ago, anticoagulants were given to everyone after a heart attack. Today, anticoagulants are not prescribed as a matter of course. They are used only under specific circumstances. For example, if a person has a history of blood clots in the veins or lungs, or if a person shows signs of an excessive tendency toward clotting.

Anticoagulants should not be taken by people with severe high blood pressure, kidney failure, active stomach ulcers, or impending surgery. (If any surgery, even a tooth extraction, is planned, it is important to tell the dentist you are taking an anticoagulant.)

Possible Side Effects: If anticoagulants are too strong, bleeding can occur. There may be internal bleeding or profuse bleeding, even from a minor cut. Symptoms of this bleeding include:

· black and blue spots without having been bruised
· nosebleeds
· blood in the urine
· red or black blood in the stools (from bleeding in the stomach and intestines)
· headaches (due to bleeding in the brain)

Other possible side effects of anticoagulants include skin rash, nausea, cramps, diarrhea, and fever.

If any side effects from anticoagulants occur, you should stop the medicine immediately and call your doctor. He will probably prescribe other drugs which can stop this bleeding.

Propranolol (Trade Name: Inderal)

Propranolol is a newer drug, often prescribed for the relief of angina when nitroglycerin alone is not sufficient. Many times it is given along with long-acting nitroglycerin.

Propranolol slows the pulse rate and allows the heart to beat more gently. It permits the heart to work less.

How It Looks: Propranolol comes in orange, 10 mg tablets; green, 40 mg tablets; and yellow, 80 mg tablets. It may be taken

Be aware:

Other medicines—particularly aspirin and aspirin-containing products—if taken along with an anticoagulant can increase the risk of bleeding. The following drugs contain aspirin: Dristan, Darvon compound, Fiorinal, Alka-Seltzer (regular formula), Anacin, Bufferin, Empirin, Excedrin, Midol, Sine-off, Triaminicin.

Drugs like phenobarbital and other sedatives can interfere with anticoagulant action. Therefore, if taking an anticoagulant, never take any drug, even a seemingly harmless one, before checking with your physician.

several times a day. In case of emergency, it can also be given by injection.

What It Does: Propranolol makes the heart function better with the oxygen it is receiving. It does this in a special way. Adrenaline is a strong heart stimulant. The body always has a small amount of adrenaline in the blood stream. Propranolol makes the heart less responsive to adrenaline. The heart pumps more slowly, thus it does not have to work as hard. Because it pumps more slowly and less forcefully, it needs less oxygen. A heart that needs less oxygen is less likely to have angina which is brought on by a shortage of oxygen.

Who Should Take It: Propranolol is used for people with angina or high blood pressure. It is also useful in decreasing a rapid pulse rate in people with an overactive thyroid. The amount of the drug varies from person to person. When the drug is taken, the pulse rate usually slows but the dosage is adjusted so the pulse does not go below fifty to fifty-five beats per minute.

Possible Side Effects: Propranolol is often used in combination with other heart drugs. The precise combination is a matter of delicate medical management since side effects can occur. These side effects, and what can be done about them follow. If any side effects occur, it is essential to notify your doctor immediately.

Possible Side Effects	What Your Doctor May Advise
Short-winded, cough a lot at night	Readjust dosage and add digitalis or a diuretic
Numbness of the hands, lightheadedness, constipation, blue spots on the skin, weakness	Adjust dosage
Nausea, vomiting, depression, hair loss, diarrhea	Stop the drug

Be aware:

1. It is very important to understand that propranolol cannot be discontinued abruptly. An abrupt stoppage can cause the heart's need for oxygen to rise suddenly and this can bring on a heart attack. So if this drug is to be discontinued, its use should be slowly decreased over a period of several days to two weeks or more. Of course, it must be done under the close supervision of a physician.

2. If you are going to have surgery of any kind, be sure that the surgeon knows you are using propranolol. Its presence in the body could complicate the effects of anesthesia. Some doctors recommend discontinuing the drug gradually and then stopping it completely for two days prior to surgery. Other doctors prefer to continue it to protect the heart and make other medical adjustments, if needed.

Aspirin

Believe it or not, just plain aspirin is often the main drug prescribed after a heart attack. In recent years, studies have shown that aspirin is much more than a simple pain killer. Scientists believe that aspirin works by interfering with the formation of prostaglandins. Prostaglandins contribute to tissue inflammation, the elevation of body temperature, and the clotting of the blood, among many other things.

Because of the decreased tendency of blood to clot some physicians prescribe aspirin after a heart attack. As yet, scientific studies have neither definitely confirmed nor denied this effect but studies are continuing and results should be forthcoming.

Be aware:

Aspirin should never be taken with anticoagulants since it may cause bleeding.

Vitamin E

Some doctors believe large doses of Vitamin E are beneficial to the heart. They suggest it may avoid clotting in the veins and lungs. Again, studies are continuing.

Pills Yes . . . But Remember

Unfortunately, popping pills cannot cure heart problems. It must be remembered that no drug has been discovered which cures hardening of the arteries.

Heart attacks are end stages of the long process of atherosclerosis. While drugs definitely have a role, a person's willpower —his daily commitment to a new health-minded lifestyle is the key to success. As Shakespeare wrote:

'Tis in ourselves that we are thus or thus. Our bodies are our gardens, to the which our wills are gardeners; so that if we plant nettles, or sow lettuce, set hyssop and weed up thyme, supply it with one gender of herbs, or distract it with many, either to have it sterile with idleness, or manured with industry, why, the power and corrigible authority of this lies in our wills.*

* *Othello*, Act I, Sc. 3

14. Possible Problems, Effective Treatment

A NUMBER of different problems can occur after a heart attack. Some problems are not obvious. For this reason, frequent blood tests are done in the coronary care unit. Damaged heart muscle releases enzymes into the bloodstream which can be identified and measured by blood tests. Blood tests can also uncover anemia and other problems that may be otherwise undetected and can affect the heart.

A continuous cardiogram—a constant record of the heart's electrical activity—is another way of watching for possible problems. Most importantly, the cardiogram shows abnormal heart rhythms or fibrillation. When these are recognized, prompt steps can be taken to convert this dangerous fibrillation or other irregularities into normal beating. Electrocardiogram tracings can also reveal shortages or excesses of certain elements in the blood. It can show inadequate supply of oxygen to the heart muscle. Sometimes it helps indicate the presence of a blood clot in the lung or inflammation of the pericardium.

An echocardiogram—a simple, completely painless procedure —is another commonly used method of detecting hidden problems. Often, for example, an echocardiogram can determine if there is abnormal thickness of the cardiac septum, or if a blood clot is present, or if the cardiac valves within the heart are opening and closing properly.

Many times, no problems develop, but people may misunderstand routine measures. For example, administering oxygen frightens many people and they assume a problem has developed. However, oxygen is routinely given to almost all people after a heart attack. It helps decrease the work of the heart and may even decrease the extent of the heart attack. Oxygen is given either through a small nasal tube or by face mask.

Another routine precautionary measure for all Coronary Care Unit patients is the insertion of a small needle called an IV (intravenous tube) into a vein in one arm. Through this IV, sugar and water constantly flow. If medicines are needed, they can be inserted directly into the bloodstream through the IV.

If a special problem does develop, you should be aware of it as well as the therapies most commonly used.

POSSIBLE PROBLEM: *Pain*

People who have heart attacks often suffer crushing pain in the chest, the arm, the neck, or the back.

Effective Treatment: There are a number of very effective drugs that people are given when they first get to the hospital to alleviate pain. The most well known and frequently used are morphine or Demerol. Both are narcotics, usually given intravenously. When people arrive in the coronary care unit, they are also asked to breathe oxygen which helps relieve pain. A mild sedative such as Valium is also routinely given. Nitroglycerin and related drugs are also used for the treatment of pain.

POSSIBLE PROBLEM: *Severe pain with deep breathing or lying back (pericarditis)*

Effective Treatment: Sometimes, the membrane surrounding the heart becomes inflamed. This irritation, known as pericarditis, can be quite painful, particularly when the person takes a deep breath or is lying back. A drug, indomethacin can effectively treat this problem. Corticosteroids are also used for this. Aspirin is generally not used in the treatment of heart-attack-related pericarditis.

POSSIBLE PROBLEM: *Irregular heartbeat—too fast (tachycardia)*

Effective Treatment: As explained earlier, people who have heart attacks frequently have problems associated with the electrical system of the heart. Three forms of therapy are used to treat this problem. First, antiarrhythmic drugs are given intravenously or orally. Some of these drugs are lidocaine (Xylocaine), procaina-

mide (Pronestyl), quinidine, propranolol (Inderal), diphenylhy-
dantoin (Dilantin) and digoxin (Lanoxin). They are used alone
or in combination. If these drugs do not work, defibrillation or
cardioversion may be used. In defibrillation, a large electric shock
is given. This is an emergency procedure. Cardioversion, a procedure for less severe abnormalities of heartbeat, provides smaller
shocks in a particular phase of the cardiac cycle.

POSSIBLE PROBLEM: *Irregular heart beat—too slow*

Effective Treatment: Damage to the electrical system within
the heart often causes the heartbeat to slow markedly. In such
cases, a pacemaker is inserted.

Some pacemakers are permanent. These are needed when the
damage is beyond the point of healing or the likelihood of slow-
beat recurrence is high. Permanent pacemakers are inserted by a
surgeon directly under the skin of the chest. The small operation
takes about an hour and is done under local anaesthesia.

Other pacemakers are temporary. They work through a device
outside the body with wires placed into the right auricle and/or
ventricle via a vein, in a fashion similar to inserting an intravenous
tube. They are needed only for a few days until the abnormality
has been corrected.

A number of different permanent pacemakers are available;
all are quite reliable and are inserted during a brief operation. They
consist of a wire and a "pulse generator." All are run on batteries
and must be periodically replaced every three or more years depending on the energy source.

People with pacemakers can lead normal lives. They can swim,
play tennis, and drive.

Today, most pacemakers work "on demand." This means that
as long as the heart rate remains at a prescribed level, the pacemaker remains inactive. If the person's heart rate drops below
that level, the pacemaker immediately begins sending impulses
to promote the beat.

In most cases, pacemakers improve the person's sense of well-
being. People do not have to worry about malfunctioning. Even if
the pacemaker has a technical problem it is rarely life-endangering,
since most people have some function left in the electrical system
of their hearts. Special devices are available to check on a pace-

maker's function after it has been inserted. If a problem is detected, another small operation can be done and it can be replaced.

Be aware:

If faintness, dizziness, or rapid heart action are experienced, one should immediately contact a physician or go to a hospital emergency room for evaluation of the pacemaker.

POSSIBLE PROBLEM: *Congestive heart failure (shortness of breath)*

Effective Treatment: It is not uncommon for people to develop congestive heart failure during the first few days or weeks after a heart attack.

Congestive heart failure does not mean the heart is not pumping. Rather, the heart contracts a little less efficiently. Each time it contracts, it pumps some blood but some remains behind. This may lead to a fluid build-up in the lungs, tissue spaces, ankles, and perhaps abdomen.

A number of drugs are used to treat congestive heart failure. These include digitalis, which strengthens the heartbeat, and diuretics, which remove excess fluid from the lungs and body. Drugs such as hydralazine and nitrates are also used to lessen the heart's work.

POSSIBLE PROBLEM: *Blood clots*

Effective Treatment: For some people, blood clots occur either during a heart attack or immediately after. These blood clots can travel from leg veins to the lungs. Anticoagulant drugs are given for this problem. The most common is heparin which can be given only by injection. Oral blood thinners are also used. The most commonly prescribed is warfarin sodium (Coumadin). It can be taken by mouth and is usually given for a number of months.

POSSIBLE PROBLEM: *Severe breathing difficulties*

Effective Treatment: Rarely, people experience severe breathing difficulties during recovery from a heart attack. In such instances, a tube is inserted into the person's windpipe. This is connected to a respirator which pumps air into the lungs at regular intervals to help the person to breathe.

POSSIBLE PROBLEM: *Intolerable anginal pain*

Effective Treatment: Coronary bypass surgery—also called coronary revascularization—detours diseased arteries, brings more blood to the heart muscle and thus relieves this severe pain. Although this procedure has become very popular—more than 70,000 were performed last year—a person should not rush into bypass surgery blindly.

Is Surgery the Answer?

When angina pain keeps a person from enjoying his life and even working, bypass surgery *can* be the answer, but it is always advisable to try conventional medical treatments first. (The exception is if the left main coronary artery is blocked, or if there is severe multi-vessel disease, then surgeons usually operate immediately.)

Bypass surgery has great value for some people after a heart attack, sometimes even before a heart attack. But it is a serious operation and not advisable for everyone. Here are some facts you should know.

What Is Coronary Artery Bypass Surgery?

Bypass surgery is a means of bypassing clogged arteries which are interfering with blood supply to the heart. It is called a "bypass operation" because surgeons graft a piece of vein—removed usually from the patient's leg. This new vessel creates a new blood supply route to the heart muscle.

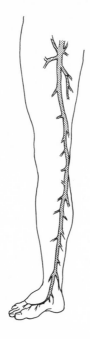

SAPHENOUS VEIN

During a bypass procedure, the saphenous vein from the leg is removed and sewn into the heart. This does not affect leg function at all.

How Much Does It Cost?

There are long waiting lists for the operation despite a price tag of about $12,500. Of course, costs vary according to institution, location, surgeon, and the person's condition before and after surgery. Much of the cost may be reimbursed through health insurance.

What Kind of Results Can Be Expected from Bypass Surgery?

Most patients report feeling vastly better following bypass surgery. A typical patient, a fifty-two-year-old book editor who had suffered from progressively worsening chest pains for three years and who had severe narrowing in three major coronary arteries, describes how he now feels (eight months following his operation).

"I probably have not felt this good since my twenties. I had forgotten what it was like to walk briskly for five or six blocks without feeling breathless or having chest pains. I can only describe it as having a new lease on life."

Is Bypass Surgery Done Even Before a Heart Attack?

Many times. With the onset of new angina or "unstable" angina—a serious form of angina that often mimics a heart attack because of its intensity—bypass surgery is frequently recommended if drug therapy fails.

Is Bypass Right for Everyone?

Doctors consider many factors before recommending bypass surgery: the person's age and overall condition, the severity of the heart disease, and the success of other medical treatments. After heart attacks, people should be treated with medicines, if possible. If these do not work, however, surgery may be recommended. It is usually the treatment of choice for people with disabling chest pains that drugs cannot control or people who have certain types of critical artery blockages.

What Tests Are Done Before a Decision Is Made to Operate?

Before operating, the surgeons must be able to see where the coronary arteries are blocked. To do this, a procedure called an *angiocardiography* or *cardiac catheterization* is done. This involves injecting X-ray-sensitive material through a catheter—a long flexible tube that can be threaded directly into the heart from an arm or groin artery—and then using X rays to follow the movement of this opaque substance in the coronary arteries. In this way, doctors can pinpoint the areas that are narrowed and determine the extent of the disease.

Who Does Cardiac Catheterization?

This minor operation, done under local anesthesia by a cardiologist, takes about an hour.

Is It Safe?

It is a basically safe procedure, but there are flaws. The major complications are thrombosis at the insertion site, a heart attack or arrhythmia secondary to catheter trauma, and death. Mortality rates of one per 1,000 have been reported. High-grade main stem left coronary artery disease appears to increase the risk of death and therefore many angiographers routinely flush dye into the left coronary sinus to rule out left main stem disease before beginning the catheter insertion.

Despite these risks, coronary angiography is recommended by most doctors for evaluation of coronary artery disease in patients being considered for surgery and in patients with unusual, puzzling, or atypical chest pain.

Is Bypass Surgery the Same as Open-Heart Surgery?

Open-heart surgery refers to surgery performed on the opened heart while blood is diverted through a heart-lung machine. Bypass surgery is an open-heart procedure.

During bypass surgery, the person's heart is opened and the heart is stopped. During this time, the person is connected to the

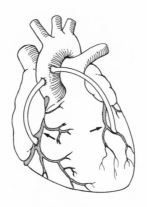

BYPASS GRAFTS

Coronary artery bypass operations are the commonest major operation in the U.S. today. In this procedure, grafts connect the coronary arteries with the aorta, creating a new passageway to the heart muscle.

heart-lung machine which temporarily takes over the work of both the heart and lungs. It removes carbon dioxide from the blood, adds oxygen, and pumps blood through the body.

How Is the Surgery Done?

The idea of bypass surgery is much like creating a road detour around an obstruction. First, an incision is made in the leg and a length of vein is removed. At the same time, the person's chest is opened.

The vein is then tested and prepared. Before the vein's insertion in the heart, the person is attached to the heart-lung machine. This gives the surgeon a quieter work space. The vein is then attached to a point beyond the blocked area. The other end is attached to the aorta. Other bypasses are done in the same way.

The operation takes three to six hours. When the bypassing is completed, the patient is disconnected from the heart-lung machine. It is then possible to get a measure, through instrumentation, of the improved blood flow to the heart's muscle. When, at last, the patient's chest is closed, he or she goes to the recovery room. After surgery, the patient then spends several days in the intensive care unit for monitoring. Many people stay in the hospital only ten days and are back at work in four to six weeks. Of course, this varies from person to person.

Does Bypass Cure Atherosclerosis?

No. The underlying atherosclerosis process may continue to narrow other coronary arteries and even these new passageways.

Is Bypass Performed in Most Hospitals?

Most large hospitals, particularly those associated with medical schools, perform open-heart surgery. However, some surgeons and institutions have much better records than others.

Patients should ask the surgeon how often he does this particular type of heart operation. Ideally, he and his surgery team should operate at least three times a week and there should be an experienced postoperative team familiar with handling heart surgery patients. Don't be afraid to ask how much experience your surgeon has and how often a death has occurred after these operations. You have a right to know such facts.

Are the Results Permanent?

While many people rave about the remarkable results, these are not necessarily permanent. About 80 percent of the grafts remain open one to five years after the operation. A very strong warning is needed to prevent feelings of false security. Bypass surgery is *not* a cure for atherosclerosis. Within a few years, the new grafts may also become narrowed or blocked with fatty deposits. This is why patients who undergo bypass surgery must also adjust their lifestyle and reduce the risk factors.

Will Bypass Surgery Prevent Another Heart Attack?

It might delay or even prevent a heart attack in some patients but there is no guarantee of this.

Will Bypass Surgery Help the Person Live Longer?

Some studies have found that patients with certain types of blockages, for example, severe narrowing of the main left coronary artery, or three-vessel involvement, do live longer. But for most people, surgery does not extend life. However, it often makes everyday living more enjoyable.

How Safe Are These Operations?

This is a serious operation. The risk of death varies from less than 2 percent to more than 20 percent, depending upon the surgeon and the person's condition.

During or immediately after the operation, about 10 percent of patients may experience a heart attack despite expert medical attention. These attacks are generally smaller in size, occurring as they do in a controlled situation.

However, the vast majority of operations are done safely. The grafts are able to supply the heart with approximately the same amount of blood as a normal coronary artery.

Is the Operation Always Successful?

Most often, it is successful. But a person must realize that this is not always so. The vein or artery used for the bypass can occlude or close up; this occurs in some 15 to 20 percent of patients. In such cases, it usually causes a return of anginal pain, which sometimes may be worse than before surgery.

"I want a bypass operation. How soon after my heart attack can I have it?"

Coronary artery bypass surgery is rarely performed on individuals who have recently had a heart attack. Usually two to three months are allowed to elapse between a heart attack and cardiac surgery.

"I am short of breath all the time. Can bypass surgery help me?"

Shortness of breath is usually a symptom of heart failure (failure of the heart to pump enough blood).

Generally, bypass surgery is not effective in improving heart failure and rarely relieves shortness of breath. In addition, bypass surgery presents greater risks for people with significant heart failure.

The Emotional Element

Surgery is not only a shock to the body, it involves emotional upheaval as well. However, most people feel they have no choice. As one fifty-five-year-old woman put it, "Frankly, I just didn't think that much about it. I knew I had to do it. When I read about the operation, I was basically unmoved. I just felt it was something that had to be done."

For families, it is extremely difficult. "It was a worse ordeal for my husband," this woman recounted, "I was the patient, lying in bed, but my husband was the one who looked bad and was aging."

It is important to be aware that immediately after surgery, people do not look well. This woman's twenty-five-year-old daughter said, "When my mother came out of surgery, it was the most horrid sight. Her face was somehow distorted from the tubes and she looked awful. I wasn't prepared for that. But two days later, she looked remarkably well—almost back to normal."

Relax—Have a Drink

Problems after a heart attack—whether medical or emotional —bring tension. Alcohol may be harmful to the heart, but doctors recognize that tension can often be more harmful. So cardiologists say alcohol is fine in moderation. This means that one medium-strength cocktail or one glass of beer or wine a day are probably safe for most people after they have recovered from a heart attack. For more on this subject, see page 211.

Medical and emotional problems can complicate an already difficult situation. By knowing about them, however, you can follow your physician's advice with greater understanding and confidence. And, remember, with today's medical advances the quality of life after a heart attack—even a complicated one—is remarkably better than ever before.

I5. A Look Ahead

THERE is a tremendous amount of intriguing and exciting research being done around the world to conquer heart problems. In very recent years, heart disease mortality has declined strikingly. Almost certainly, further progress can be expected—some of it quite likely within a very few years.

This chapter will explore these future solutions—some may prove of little practical use but undoubtedly many will be immensely rewarding.

The Artificial Heart

As many as 50,000 people a year would be immediate candidates for an artificial heart if such a device were available. Research has been under way since 1974 both in the United States and Russia to produce an artificial heart.

Several prototype artificial hearts have been developed. One, for example, is made of two air-driven pumps that would replace the ventricles or pumping chambers. They would be attached to the remnants of the upper chambers of the heart. The heartbeat would be triggered by pacemaking cells in the remnant of the upper right atrium.

Artificial hearts have been implanted in laboratory animals, even calves, with success. In the United States and Russia, in 1976, artificial hearts were implanted into calves and were kept going for several hours without mechanical failure. An American team led by Dr. William J. Kolff (the inventor of the artificial kidney machine) has implanted artificial hearts in calves twenty-five times with success. In one calf experiment the heart worked for twenty-one days and the calf was even able to exercise on a tread-mill.

Energy sources for the artificial heart have been a problem. Current models get their power from consoles outside the body; obviously, an implantable power source is needed. Various possibilities are under study, including some devices that convert body heat to electricity and others that convert body motion to electricity. Plutonium 238 is also being studied because its low weight and power potential are attractive, but radioactivity is a problem. Belt-worn battery packs are another possibility.

Finding a suitable material for the artificial heart is another problem for scientists. This is not an easy task since the material must not cause body rejection, it must not cause allergic or toxic reactions, and it must be strong enough to withstand stress for many years.

A totally artificial heart will need two pumping units: a right side for pumping to the lungs and a left side for pumping to the body. It is hoped that success may be near, since one-sided left ventricular assist devices are already being successfully used in open-heart operations.

Recently, a double-sided device was successfully used for the first time in a human in Switzerland when a man's heart could not pump effectively after surgery. For two days, this device supported circulation until the patient's heart resumed efficient pumping.

Artificial Blood

Another exciting area of research concerns artificial blood. This blood substitute would mix and dissolve into human blood and carry oxygen just as real blood does. However, man-made blood would not have the tendency to cause atherosclerosis as normal blood does. With artificial blood, people would have the benefits of real blood without the drawbacks. In addition, artificial blood could be used in heart surgery in situations where real blood is unavailable.

Heart Transplantation

Today and for the near future, when all other medical and surgical measures have failed, transplantation seems the best solution to end-stage heart disease or severely disabling angina. Transplant recipients include a professional bowler, a television reporter, a doctor, and many others.

To be a candidate for a transplant, a patient must be desperately ill—his condition must be so serious that he or she is limited to a bed-to-chair existence and no further medical or surgical treatment is possible. Most transplant patients are under fifty years of age and all have a clinically estimated life span of less than six months without heart transplantation.

Do transplants work? According to a Stanford report, heart transplantation "clearly improves the quality of life in surviving patients." Many patients, once bedridden or severely limited, return to "normal activity status"—meaning no symptoms even with vigorous activity. But mortality is high.

At the world center for transplantation, Stanford University Medical Center in Palo Alto, California, directed by Dr. Norman Shumway, the one-year survival rate is now 70 percent compared with 42 percent ten years ago. Of 150 patients that received heart transplants between January 1978 and August 1979, sixty-two lived to the end of this period.

Most doctors feel an artificial heart will eventually be preferable to transplantation. It will eliminate the problems of rejection and antirejection drugs whose effects on the body can be devastating. For now, transplantation is an answer. Many people who undoubtedly would have died are still alive. Indeed, a Frenchman, now alive more than ten years after his transplant, outlived his transplant surgeon!

The three main problems with transplants are donors, rejection, and infection. Donors are usually young people with healthy hearts who die in accidents. Organ banks, with the aid of computers, now match suitable donors with recipients around the world. Recently, two New York kidneys were transplanted less than a day later into a Moscow recipient. Some day, the same will be done for hearts.

Rejection and infection—it's a maxim among those working on organ transplants that recipients get one or the other. Better methods of matching donor hearts to patients and refinement of methods of combating rejection have somewhat reduced the rejection problem. It is no longer a major cause of death.

Susceptibility to infection, however, has remained an inevitable side effect of antirejection drugs. Infections are becoming a major cause of death in long-term survivors.

Cost is another factor. In late 1977, an average hospital stay of seventy-two days was required, and inpatient costs for the operation and early post-operative care averaged $36,130 per patient.

It is hoped that in the future, problems of donor availability, rejection, infection, and cost can be solved so transplantation can become more practical on a large scale.

Echocardiography: Insight Through Sound

Just over ten years ago, the clinical introduction of echocardiography revolutionized the practice of cardiology. Echocardiography displays sound patterns correlating with the motion, speed, and thickness of moving heart structures. From these patterns the volumes and pumping efficiency of the cardiac chambers can be obtained with considerable accuracy, preventing the need for more costly, and sometimes riskier, cardiac catheterization and angiography. Today, these signals are processed by computer and actual cardiac images result. This technique is called "real time" or "two-dimensional echocardiography." At present, floppy valve tissue, atrial and ventricular septal defects, and abnormal muscle thickenings are some of the heart defects that can be seen with echocardiography. In the future, perhaps doctors will be able to sound-scan coronary arteries, detecting blockages before they become problems. Already, sound is being used to detect early atherosclerotic plaque formations in the arteries of the neck leading to the brain.

Radioisotopes: A Touch of "Star Wars"

Current work with radioisotopes is another fascinating research frontier. Today, techniques using small doses of radioisotopes that emit gamma radiation are used to measure the heart function—during pumping or systole and during rest or diastole. This is often done at a regular exercise test. Called a *thallium perfusion test* or a stress and rest scan, a small dose of radioactive thallous chloride is injected into a small arm vein at the point of maximum exercise. Gamma camera pictures are taken. About four hours later, at rest, these pictures are repeated. Areas of "underperfusion" or defects can sometimes be seen in the exercise test as compared with the rest test. These correspond to areas containing coronary artery blockages.

Today, radioisotopes are also used in exercise angiograms. This test uses bicycle exercise done while the patient is lying on a bed with attached or overhead suspended bicycle pedals. While at rest, the patient's own red blood cells are "tagged" by a tracer dose of radioisotope. Resting efficiency is determined. Then at maximum effort, pumping efficiency is measured. Any decline in pumping efficiency (ejection fraction, to a cardiologist) or poor localized contraction is a sign of cardiac disease.

On the near horizon are still more sophisticated radioisotope tests. Some new work is being done using radioactively labeled fatty acid molecules which are injected into the bloodstream. During angina, the heart may absorb these fatty acids. If so, beta radiation is emitted. Beta counting devices can then detect "sore spots" within the heart wall indicating areas of blockage. This may be the ultimate technique finally sensitive enough to detect disease in the small coronary arteries. In the future, refining of these nuclear techniques will certainly implement and may even replace cardiac catheterization.

The Question of Alcohol

The pros and cons of drinking alcohol after a heart attack have been debated for years. Traditionally, doctors believed that alcohol increased the risk of both obesity and heart attacks.

However, new research suggests that a drink a day may, in fact, keep the heart specialist away. A recent Honolulu heart study of 8,000 men reported a *lower* incidence of heart attacks in moderate drinkers. They found deaths from heart attacks were about two times as common in teetotalers than in those who had up to two beers a day. Most of those studied used only beer, so no conclusions could be made for wine or liquor in similar amounts. Interestingly those in another study who consumed a moderate amount of alcohol were found to have increased levels of high density lipoprotein—the factor thought to confer some protection against heart attack.

Indeed, a recent Cleveland Clinic study of 800 men showed that consumption of more than four drinks a day gave consistently higher HDL levels, thus more heart protection.

Still, the question of alcohol after a heart attack remains controversial. In the future, this will hopefully be better understood.

New Drugs: New Hope

Digitalis strengthens the failing heart but the drug still has many problems. For example, there is a very narrow difference between a good therapeutic blood level and toxic blood levels. Even an experienced cardiologist will occasionally have a patient with high digitalis blood levels. So newer and hopefully better drugs are being studied. These include:

Aminrone: Given intravenously, this drug has the properties of both diuretics and digitalis. But side effects are still a major problem.

Calcium Blockers: Several very promising drugs (Nafedipine and Verapamil) are likely to be marketed in the near future. These may hold the key to relieving atypical angina and preventing sudden death due to coronary artery spasm.

Duloctil: Only recently, this new drug was released for patient use in Mexico. It is believed to relieve painful walking and coldness of the extremities in people with atherosclerosis.

Take an Aspirin and Don't Call the Doctor

New research suggests that aspirin may play a significant role in preventing heart attacks from occurring in the first place. Some scientists believe that someday lifelong heart attack and stroke prevention may begin with a daily or twice daily use of half an aspirin from childhood on. Interestingly, studies with monkeys show aspirin may even protect those eating high-cholesterol diets.

How does aspirin work? Probably by making the blood platelets less sticky and preventing their adherence to blood vessel walls, an important part of plaque formation. Or it may work through a hormone.

What dose should you take? It seems that platelets become slippery only when the proper dose is taken; too much aspirin may have the opposite effect. At present, the recommended dose is one or two tablets a day. Interestingly, a study at the Massachusetts General Hospital showed that aspirin lowered the incidence of floating blood clots in men after hip surgery but did not work for women.

Sex Hormones and Heart Attacks

Long thought to play a role in the male's greater likelihood of having a heart attack, sex hormones have recently come under new scrutiny. For years, scientists believed it was the male's testosterone that somehow played a role in his heart attack. Dr. Gerald D. Phillips and his coworkers at Columbia University's Roosevelt Hospital in New York City are now convinced that sex hormone ratios may be the crucial factor. Specifically, their studies show high estriol concentrations in males are associated with heart attacks. This means a higher estriol to testosterone ratio. (Usually men have some female hormones but in far lower concentrations than females.) This new theory may drastically alter the thrust of heart attack research and resistance will undoubtedly be encountered. Should this work be confirmed, however, it would not be difficult to normalize the hormone ratios to prevent heart attacks in men.

Vitamin E

Vitamin E has long been the subject of cardiac research but has come under new attention recently. As far back as 1936, Vitamin E research showed that Vitamin E deficiency promoted myocardial scarring.

In 1947, work on the relationship of Vitamin E to retarding arterial lesions started. Recently research was published showing improvement in exercise walking tolerance for people with arterial disease of the leg when given 300 mg of Vitamin E a day. In some people arterial flow increased over 34 percent. Vitamin E has also been shown to eliminate nighttime leg and foot cramps. Response can occur within a week. On discontinuing medication, the symptoms promptly recur. What does all this have to do with heart attacks? Leg problems are vascular and so is a heart attack. Vitamin E is believed to inhibit platelet aggregation in ways similar to aspirin but research is far from conclusive. Further research is needed to explore the possible usefulness of large daily doses of Vitamin E in preventing vascular problems.

Is There a Long-Life Diet for the Heart?

Dr. Nathan Pritikin adamantly believes there is. His LFC (low fat and cholesterol) diet limits fats to less than 15 percent of total daily calories and cholesterol to less than 100 mg a day, and omits all simple carbohydrates such as molasses, sugar, and honey. Dr. Pritikin calls the disease that results from excessively high levels of cholesterol, lipids, and triglycerides "lipo toxemia" ("lipo" for fat, "toxemia" for poisoning).

His results have been inspiring. Converts to his diet and way of life exude happiness and seeming health. There are people reportedly too ill to have bypass surgery—people plagued by angina at the slightest provocation—who have become asymptomatic on the Pritikin program. These outstanding results cannot be ignored. Although controlled studies are still under way, it seems obvious to many cardiologists and patients alike that one wave of the future may be a heart-tailored diet.

Today, heart attacks still baffle physicians, and many areas of patient care are controversial even among experts. The magnitude of the problem is immense—almost immeasurable. In a recent year, almost a million lives were cut off by heart and blood vessel disease, about thirty billion dollars of income was unearned, and over fifty million man-days of work were wasted.

Progress has been made, and it is encouraging to realize that deaths are decreasing. Today, more people survive heart attacks than die from them. The quality of life for most heart attack victims is better than ever before.

With the dynamic research currently under way, it is realistic to hope that within our lifetime, heart disease will be America's *former* rather than present Number One health problem.

APPENDIX A Danger Signs: When to Call Your Doctor

Everyone should know these warning signs. If a heart attack strikes, there is no time for delay. The common symptoms are:

- a heavy, squeezing pain or discomfort in the center of the chest which may last for several minutes (sharp, stabbing pains do not usually mean heart disease). It may be intense or it may resemble indigestion.
- pain which may radiate to the shoulder, arm, neck, or jaw
- nausea, vomiting
- difficulty breathing
- sweating
- anxiety
- palpitations

Sometimes symptoms go away and then recur.

If someone develops these symptoms, call the doctor or emergency number right away (in many communities, the number is 911). If you have trouble getting help by phone, get to a hospital emergency room at once. Minutes and even seconds can be crucial.

APPENDIX B *Special* Heart Tests

After a heart attack special heart tests are usually done to provide a more detailed picture of the heart's condition. The most common procedures are reviewed below. By understanding them, you will realize they are neither mysterious nor frightening. Most are simple, short, and painless. Some are done in the doctor's office, others in a hospital or clinic. (Most do not require staying overnight.)

Electrocardiogram. The electrocardiogram (ECG or EKG) gives a tracing on graph paper of the electrical activity of the heart. It can reveal arrhythmias—irregular heart rhythms. It also shows the kind, extent, and location of the damage caused by the heart attack. An EKG is most often taken while the person is lying down. This is sometimes called a resting EKG.

Chest X Ray. A chest X ray is created when an X-ray machine briefly sends minute amounts of radiation through the chest and onto a photographic plate. When developed, this "photo" will show the internal chest structures: ribs, lungs, heart, and blood vessels. After a heart attack, chest X rays are useful in revealing enlargement of the heart— very often one sign of a chronic heart problem—and in detailing the circulatory system of the lungs.

Blood Tests. Blood tests are extremely useful in evaluating heart functions. Enzymes (chemicals used by the heart to function normally) are released from the damaged heart tissue into the bloodstream. Abnormal levels of these enzymes (CPK, SGOT, LDH) can be measured in a blood sample.

Blood tests can also reveal abnormally high levels of blood fats (lipids). These lead to atherosclerotic deposits and heart attacks.

Blood tests are also important in detecting abnormal glucose or blood sugar levels, that may indicate diabetes mellitus, which increases the risk of heart and blood vessel disease.

Various blood tests are also used to regulate heart drug dosage.

Exercise Electrocardiogram. Sometimes called a stress test, this is an EKG recorded while the patient is exercising—usually walking or jogging on a treadmill or pedaling on a stationary bicycle or perhaps walking up and down a step. An exercise EKG can sometimes reveal heart ailments which show up only when the heart is under physical stress. For this reason, it should be done only in the presence of a physician.

Fluoroscopy. Like chest X rays, fluoroscopy involves visualizing internal organs by means of radiation. Instead of looking at still X-ray pictures, however, the physician can watch the heart shadow in motion. Fluoroscopy can be useful in revealing irregularities in heart chamber size or function and calcification (hardening of valves and vessels). It is often used with other procedures, for example, cardiac catheterization. (Your doctor may be able to do fluoroscopy in his or her office but chances are it will be done in a hospital setting.)

Phonocardiography. Phonocardiography is the recording of heart sounds by microphones placed on the chest which are connected to sensitive recording equipment. For a visual record, the output signals from the microphone can be automatically traced on graph paper. This is used most often to diagnose heart murmurs.

Echocardiography. Echocardiography is a technique by which pulses of sound are transmitted into the chest by a small device placed on the skin. (This is a harmless, high frequency sound which cannot be heard by human ears.) The different echoes returning from the heart are then electronically plotted and recorded. These signals create a graphic image of the the heart and blood vessels. This can provide useful information, such as the size, shape, and motion of the heart chambers and great vessels and the motion of the heart valves.

Angiocardiography by Cardiac Catheterization. "Angiocardiography" means visualization of the heart, its vessels and chambers. Sometimes the shorter term "angiography" is used. When the technique is used only for arteries, it may be called "arteriography."

One method of angiocardiography is by cardiac catheterization. A catheter is a thin, flexible tube which can be guided into body organs. A cardiac catheter is made of material to which blood may not adhere, such as woven plastic. It is inserted into a vein or artery (usually of a leg or an arm) and gently threaded to the heart while the doctor views its progress with a fluoroscope.

Blood samples from the heart can be withdrawn through the catheter for laboratory chemical analysis. Blood pressure in the individual heart chambers, across heart valves, or in the great vessels can be measured as well as the rate at which the blood is being pumped by the heart.

Cardiac catheterization requires hospitalization (for two or three days) as it requires a local anesthetic and observation after the test.

Angiocardiography by Radioisotopic Scanning. The heart, its vessels and chambers can also be visualized by radioistotopic scanning. This involves injection into the bloodstream of certain radioisotopes, substances which are slightly radioactive for a short period of time (a few hours or so). Using a sensitive device known as a gamma scanner, a physician can record the tiny amounts of radioactivity emitted as the radioisotope circulates through the heart chambers and great vessels. These records help in evaluating blood supply to the heart, heart size, amount of blood pumped per beat, and the extent of any heart muscle damage.

Be informed:

These are the procedures most commonly used to diagnose heart problems; if other conditions are suspected in the course of an examination, other tests may be required.

GLOSSARY

This glossary contains a selection of words and phrases commonly used in the heart field. They were chosen on the basis of frequency of use and the possibility of general unfamiliarity or ambiguity.

ANEURYSM   A ballooning-out of the wall of a vein or artery or chamber of the heart due to a weakening of the wall by disease.

ANGINA PECTORIS   An episode of temporary chest pain due to inadequate oxygen to the heart muscle. The pain lasts only a few minutes and is relieved by rest or nitroglycerin.

ANGIOGRAM   An X-ray study in which dye is injected through small plastic tubes into the heart or blood vessels. The X-ray photos reveal abnormalities in the heart or blood vessels.

ANOXIA   Literally, no oxygen. This occurs when the blood supply (and hence the oxygen supply) to a part of the body is completely cut off and causes the death of the affected tissue. For example, in a heart attack, a specific area of heart muscle will die when the blood supply to that area is blocked.

ANTICOAGULANT   A drug which delays clotting of the blood. It can prevent new clots from forming or existing clots from enlarging but cannot dissolve an existing clot. Examples are heparin and coumarin derivatives.

ANTIHYPERTENSIVE DRUGS   Drugs which are used to control high blood pressure (hypertension).

  The most commonly given are diuretics which promote the elimination of excess fluids. Other types lower pressure by affecting the dilation of arteries. Still others slow the heartbeat by decreasing the force of the heart's contractions.

ANXIETY   A feeling of apprehension.

AORTA   The largest artery which carries blood away from the heart to the rest of the body.

AORTIC INSUFFICIENCY   An improper closing of the valve between the

219

aorta and the left ventricle of the heart permitting a backflow of blood.

AORTIC VALVE   Valve at the junction of the aorta and the left ventricle. It allows the blood to flow from the heart into the aorta and prevents backflow.

ARRHYTHMIA   Any variation from the normal heart rhythm.

ARTERIOSCLEROSIS   A group of diseases characterized by thickening and loss of elasticity of artery walls so that less than normal amounts of blood are able to flow through. See *atherosclerosis*.

ARTERY   A blood vessel that carries nourishing, oxygen-rich blood from the heart to the other organs of the body.

ATHEROSCLEROSIS   A kind of arteriosclerosis in which the inner layer of the artery wall is made thick and irregular by deposits of fatty substances. These fatty deposits decrease the diameter of the vessel, thus decreasing blood flow.

ATRIAL FIBRILLATION   A chaotic irregular beating of the atria, resulting from an irregular and accelerated heartbeat. This can be controlled by drugs.

ATRIAL SEPTUM   The wall dividing the left and right upper chambers of the heart (the atria).

ATRIOVENTRICULAR NODE.   A small mass of fibers between the upper chambers of the heart. It is a channel for electrical impulses which regulate the rhythm of the heartbeat.

ATRIUM   The upper chambers of the heart (also called auricles). The right atrium receives unoxygenated blood from the body. The left atrium receives oxygenated blood from the lungs. These chambers fill the pumping chambers (ventricles) below.

ATROPINE   A drug used to treat, among other things, an abnormally slow heart rate.

AUSCULTATION   The act of listening to sounds within the body, usually with a stethoscope.

AUTONOMIC NERVOUS SYSTEM   Sometimes called the involuntary nervous system. The nerves of this system regulate tissues and functions not normally under conscious control (heartbeat, blood pressure, etc.).

BLOOD PRESSURE   The force the flowing blood exerts against the artery walls. Two pressures are usually measured:

1. The systolic pressure occurs each time the heart contracts and pumps blood into the aorta.
2. The diastolic pressure occurs when the heart relaxes and refills with blood.

CAPILLARIES   The tiniest blood vessels.

CARBON MONOXIDE   A poisonous gas inhaled during smoking. Carbon monoxide combines with elements in the blood and prevents them from carrying their normal amount of oxygen.

CARDIAC   Pertaining to the heart. Sometimes refers to a person who has heart disease.

CARDIAC ARREST   Cessation of the heartbeat. As a result, blood pressure drops abruptly and the circulation of blood ceases. Until recently, this was always fatal. Today, the heart can be stimulated to start beating again under certain circumstances.

CARDIAC CATHETERIZATION   The process of introducing a thin, flexible tube into a vein or artery and guiding it into the heart for purposes of examination or treatment.

CARDIAC OUTPUT   The amount of blood pumped by the heart per minute.

CARDIOLOGIST   A specialist in the diagnosis and treatment of heart disease.

CARDIOLOGY   The study of the heart and its functions.

CARDIOPULMONARY RESUSCITATION (CPR)   An emergency measure to maintain a person's breathing and heartbeat in the event these functions suddenly stop.

CARDIOVERSION   The delivery of an electric shock to the heart that stops a cardiac arrhythmia (abnormal heartbeat).

CATHETER   A thin, flexible tube which can be guided into body organs. A cardiac catheter is made of plastic to which blood will not adhere and is inserted into a vein or artery (usually of an arm or leg) and gently threaded into the heart. Its progress can be watched on a fluoroscope.

CHOLESTEROL   A fatty substance, essential to life, that is a normal part of the blood. High levels of cholesterol, however, predispose individuals to atherosclerosis and heart attacks.

COLLATERAL CIRCULATION   Circulation of the blood through nearby smaller vessels when a main vessel has been blocked.

CONGENITAL HEART DISEASE   Heart disease due to abnormal construction of the heart that has existed since birth.

CONGESTIVE HEART FAILURE   A condition in which the heart is unable to pump proper amounts of blood.

Heart failure is often congestive because loss of pumping power by the heart leads to "congestion" in the body tissues; that is, fluid accumulates in the abdomen and legs and/or in the lungs. This condition can be treated by drugs or in some cases by surgery.

CORONARY   Frequently used as an informal term to mean a heart attack.

CORONARY ARTERIES   Arteries which carry blood to the heart muscle.

CORONARY ARTERIOGRAPHY   An X-ray technique to obtain pictures of the coronary arteries.

CORONARY ARTERY DISEASE   Heart disease caused by a narrowing of the coronary arteries which can eventually cause inadequate blood supply to part of the wall. Also called coronary heart disease, or ischemic heart disease.

CORONARY BYPASS SURGERY   Surgery to improve the blood supply to the heart muscle when this supply has been reduced due to narrowed coronary arteries.

CORONARY INSUFFICIENCY   A condition which occurs whenever coronary arteries do not provide adequate oxygen to one part of the heart. This may produce chest pain or a heart attack.

Acute coronary insufficiency is a term used to describe chest pain that is more severe than angina pectoris but in which there is no heart muscle damage (as there would be in a heart attack).

CORONARY OCCLUSION   Another term for a heart attack. It is due to an obstruction in one of the coronary arteries which hinders blood flow to the heart muscle.

CYANOSIS   Blueness of skin caused by insufficient oxygen in the blood.

DECOMPENSATION   Inability of the heart to maintain adequate circulation usually resulting in a fluid accumulation in the tissues. A person whose heart is failing to maintain normal circulation is said to be "decompensated."

DEFIBRILLATION   The delivery of an electric shock to the heart in order to stop a life-threatening abnormal heartbeat.

DIASTOLIC   One of the two blood pressure measurements. It represents the blood pressure in the arteries during the time when the heart is filling.

DIGITALIS   A very commonly used drug that causes the heart to pump more forcefully, effectively, and regularly.

DIURETIC   A drug which promotes the excretion of urine. It is very effective in the treatment of hypertension and congestive heart failure.

DYSPNEA   The uncomfortable feeling of shortness of breath.

ECHOCARDIOGRAPHY   A painless diagnostic procedure by which pulses of sound (ultrasound) are transmitted into the body and the echoes returning from the surfaces of the heart and other structures are electronically plotted and recorded.

EDEMA   Swelling due to abnormally large amounts of fluid in the body tissues.

ELECTROCARDIOGRAM   Often referred to as ECG or EKG. A painless graphic record of heat activity.

ENDOCARDITIS   Inflammation of the inner lining of the heart (endocardium) usually due to acute rheumatic fever or an infectious agent.

EXERCISE ELECTROCARDIOGRAM   Also called stress test. An electrocardiogram taken while a person is exercising.

EXTRASYSTOLE   A contraction of the heart which occurs prematurely and interrupts the normal rhythm.

FIBRILLATION   An irregular and disorganized heartbeat. In the atrium, it is called atrial fibrillation; in the ventricles, ventricular fibrillation.

FIBRIN   An elastic, threadlike protein which forms the essential portion of a blood clot.

FLUOROSCOPY   A painless examination of the beating heart and other organs using X rays passed through the body onto a fluorescent screen. A fluoroscope is often used when doctors are trying to position catheters or pacemaker wires in the heart.

GALLOP RHYTHM   An extra heart sound which, when the heart rate is rapid enough, resembles a horse's gallop. It may or may not be significant.

HEART ATTACK   The death of a portion of heart muscle due to an obstruction in one of the coronary arteries which prevents an adequate oxygen supply to a portion of the heart.

HEART BLOCK   A condition in which the electrical impulse which travels through the heart is slowed or blocked along its path.

HEART FAILURE   A condition in which the heart is unable to pump the amount of blood required to maintain normal circulation. Heart failure often leads to "congestion" or fluid accumulation in the abdomen, legs and/or lungs (see *Congestive Heart Failure*).

HEART-LUNG MACHINE   A device connected to a patient during surgery which temporarily replaces his own heart. It pumps blood, removes carbon dioxide from the blood, and adds oxygen to the blood.

HEART MASSAGE   Also called cardiac massage. An emergency technique using compression of the heart to keep the blood pumping through the body in the event the heart stops. External heart massage involves pressing on the chest to stimulate the heart to begin beating. Internal cardiac massage is done in the operating room where the heart is directly compressed by the surgeon's hand.

HEART RATE   The number of heartbeats in a minute. The normal heart rate is between 60 and 100 beats per minute.

HEPARIN A substance which tends to prevent blood from clotting.

HYPERLIPOPROTEINEMIA The name of several blood lipid disorders involving high levels of lipoproteins in the blood. Some types of hyperlipoproteinemia are associated with the premature development of atherosclerosis and therefore an increased risk of heart attacks.

HYPERTENSION High blood pressure. Long-standing high blood pressure can cause damage to the blood vessels in the brain, heart, and kidneys. Drugs are available to lower blood pressure to normal levels.

HYPERTENSIVE A person with high blood pressure (hypertension).

HYPERTHYROIDISM A condition in which the thyroid is overactive. This may eventually lead to rapid heartbeat.

HYPOXIA Less than the normal amount of oxygen in the organs and tissues of the body.

INFARCT The tissue which dies as a result of receiving an insufficient blood supply.

ISCHEMIA A local, usually temporary, deficiency of oxygen in some part of the body, usually caused by an obstruction in the blood vessel.

ISCHEMIC HEART DISEASE Also called coronary artery disease and coronary heart disease. These are heart ailments caused by narrowing of the coronary arteries which results in a decreased blood supply to the heart.

IV Abbreviation for "intravenous." It is the placing of a needle or small plastic tube through the skin and into a vein for the purpose of administering fluids or medicines to the body.

JUGULAR VEINS Veins which return blood from the head and neck to the heart.

LIPOPROTEIN A complex consisting of lipid (fat) and protein molecules bound together. Lipids do not dissolve in the blood but circulate in the form of lipoproteins.

MALIGNANT HYPERTENSION Severe high blood pressure that may quickly cause damage to the kidney, eyes, and other organs.

MONITOR A device which records on a small television screen in the cardiac care unit and is closely observed by nurses and physicians to see if any cardiac arrhythmias are occurring.

MURMUR An extra heartbeat heard between normal heartbeats.

MYOCARDIAL INFARCTION A heart attack (see *Heart Attack*).

MYOCARDIUM The muscular wall of the heart. The thickest of the three layers of the heart wall, it lies between the inner layer (endocardium) and the outer layer (epicardium).

NEUROGENIC   Originating in the nervous system.

NITRITES   A group of chemical compounds, which cause dilation of the small blood vessels and thus lower blood pressure.

NITROGLYCERIN   A drug (one of the nitrites) which relaxes the muscles in the blood vessels. Used to relieve attacks of angina pectoris.

OCCLUSIVE   Closing or shutting off. A coronary occlusion is a closing off of a coronary artery (which supplies the heart muscle with blood).

OPEN-HEART SURGERY   Surgery performed on the opened heart.

PACEMAKER   A man-made electrical device which can regulate heartbeat. It may be placed outside the chest or within the chest wall.

PALPITATION   An abnormal heart rhythm felt by a person as a fluttering sensation.

PERICARDITIS   Inflammation of the membrane that surrounds the heart.

PERICARDIUM   A tough membrane that surrounds and protects the heart within the body.

POLYUNSATURATED FAT   A fat so constituted chemically that it is capable of absorbing additional hydrogen. These fats are substituted for saturated fat in low-cholesterol diets in an effort to lessen the hazard of fatty deposits in the blood.

PRESSOR   Tending to increase blood pressure, as "a pressor substance."

PULMONARY   Referring to the lungs.

PULMONARY ARTERY   The large artery which carries unoxygenated blood from the ventricle to the lungs.

PULMONARY EDEMA   A condition marked by an excess of fluid in the extravascular (outside the vessels) spaces in the lungs.

QUINIDINE   A medicine used to treat abnormal heartbeat rhythms.

RENAL   Referring to the kidneys.

RENAL HYPERTENSION   High blood pressure caused by damage to or disease of the kidneys or their blood vessels.

RESERPINE   A commonly used medicine which lowers blood pressure and slows heart rate.

SAPHENOUS VEIN   A large vein in the leg which is often removed and grafted onto the heart in coronary bypass surgery.

SATURATED FAT   A form of fat present in many foods, particularly those of animal origin such as meat, eggs, and whole milk. Diets rich in saturated fat are believed to be one of the causes of atherosclerosis.

SEPTAL DEFECT   An abnormal opening in the wall (septum) that normally divides the right and left sides of the heart. There are both atrial and ventricular septal defects depending on whether the upper or lower heart chambers are involved.

Sgot   A chemical released from damaged heart cells into the blood. Blood tests help to measure elevated levels of Sgot and thereby show damage to heart cells.

Sinus Rhythm   Normal heart rhythm as initiated by electrical impulses in the sinoatrial node.

Sodium   A natural element, somewhat like table salt, which is found in all plant and animal tissue. In some types of heart disease, the body retains an excess of sodium and water. Therefore, sodium intake is often restricted.

Sphygmomanometer   An instrument for measuring blood pressure. Commonly called a blood pressure cuff.

Stress Test   An exercise test. An EKG while a person is exercising to determine the heart's response to physical exertion.

Syncope   A faint. One cause for syncope can be an insufficient blood supply to the brain.

Systolic   One of the two measurements of blood pressure. Systolic blood pressure occurs when the heart is pumping. It is the higher of the two blood pressure measurements.

Tachycardia   Abnormally fast heart rate. Generally, anything over 100 beats per minute is considered a tachycardia.

Thrombosis   Formation of a blood clot within a blood vessel.

Toxic   Poisonous.

Triglyceride   A fatty substance found in the blood. Triglycerides are essential to life but elevated levels of these fat substances in the blood may contribute to the development of atherosclerosis.

Ultrasound   High-frequency sound vibrations, not audible to the human ear, used in cardiac diagnosis.

Valve   A flap of tissue which prevents backflow of blood and keeps it moving in the right direction through the heart and circulatory system.

Vasoconstrictor   Part of the involuntary nervous system, these nerves cause the arterioles to contract, narrowing the passageways and thus raising blood pressure.

Vasodilator   Part of the involuntary nervous system, these nerves cause the arterioles to relax, widening the passageways and thus lowering blood pressure.

Vein   A blood vessel that carries blood back to the heart. The blood carried in veins has given up its oxygen and is therefore darker in color.

Vena Cava   One of the two great veins which carry unoxygenated blood from the body to the right atrium of the heart. The superior vena cava brings blood from the upper part of the body (head, neck